The Forgotten Homeopathy at Home: 350 Remedies

Celebrating the natural essence of herbal remedies and their timeless role in promoting holistic wellness.

Prof. Nicole Appldon, MD.

And

Marcus Fernandios

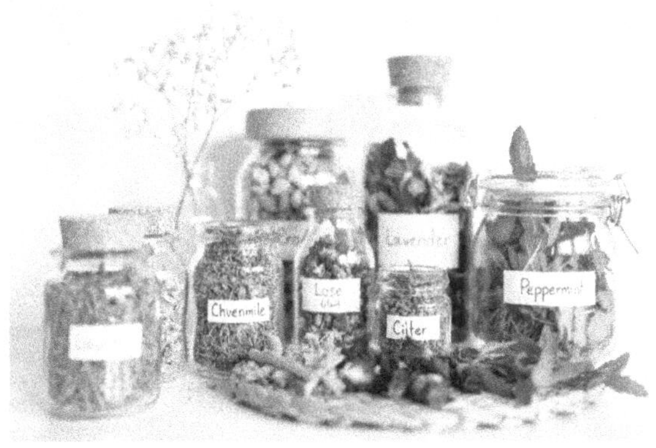

Table of Contents

About the Author

Prof. Nicole Appldon, MD, is a distinguished physician with over two decades of experience in conventional medicine and integrative wellness. Driven by a deep respect for the body's natural healing capacity, Prof. Appldon has dedicated much of her career to bridging evidence-based medical practice with time-honored herbal traditions.

Her journey into herbal medicine grew from years of clinical practice and extensive study of plant-based remedies across African and global healing systems. Through this work, she developed a profound understanding of how nature's resources can support prevention, healing, and long-term wellness when used safely and responsibly.

Prof. Appldon is a passionate advocate for holistic health education and has been actively involved in creating and guiding natural wellness initiatives that empower individuals to take an informed role in their own health. Her approach combines scientific rigor with traditional wisdom, emphasizing safety, balance, and individualized care.

Alongside her work, Prof. Appldon also acknowledges the contributions of Marcus Fernandios, a renowned homeopathy practitioner who is currently leading a homeopathy research centre in Japan. His dedication to advancing natural healing research and education reflects a shared commitment to exploring safe, responsible, and informed approaches to wellness.

Preface

The Power of Herbal Healing

Herbal medicine is one of the oldest forms of healing known to humanity. Across centuries and cultures, plants have served as powerful allies in maintaining health, preventing disease, and aiding recovery. The wisdom of herbal healing is deeply rooted in tradition, yet it continues to hold relevance in modern wellness and healthcare.

This book aims to bring together 350 carefully selected herbal remedies, drawing from rich African traditions alongside global herbal knowledge. Whether you are a curious beginner or an experienced herbalist, this compendium is designed to provide practical, clear, and safe guidance for using herbs to support your well-being.

We invite you to explore the natural pharmacy that surrounds us—plants that grow quietly but hold potent healing power. May this book inspire you to reconnect with nature and embrace a more holistic approach to health.

How to Use This Book Safely and Effectively

This compendium offers detailed information on 350 herbal remedies, including their traditional uses, preparation methods, dosages, and cautions.

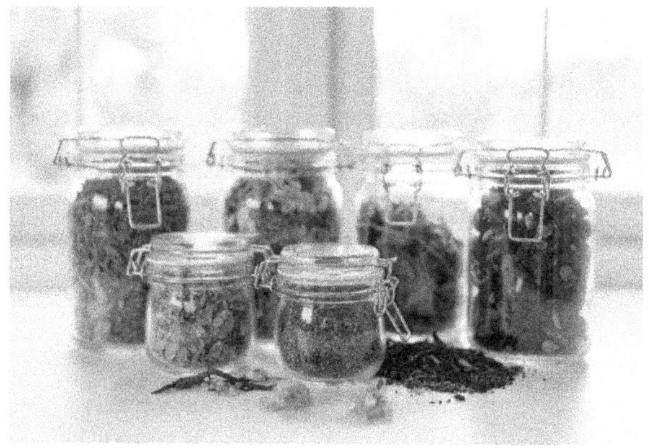

To get the most benefit and ensure safety:

- **Read carefully:** Each remedy includes detailed preparation steps and dosage guidelines. Follow these instructions closely.

- **Start slow:** When trying a new herb, begin with the lowest recommended dose to observe how your body responds.

- **Consult professionals:** Herbs can interact with medications or certain health conditions. Always talk with a qualified healthcare provider or herbalist before beginning any new treatment, especially if you are pregnant, nursing, or have chronic illnesses.

- **Avoid self-diagnosis:** Use this book as a guide, not a substitute for professional medical diagnosis or treatment.

- **Keep records:** Maintain a journal of the herbs you use, dosages, and any effects experienced. This helps track progress and avoid adverse reactions.

- **Be mindful:** Herbs are natural but potent. More is not always better; respect the recommended dosages and durations.

- **Store properly:** Keep herbs in a cool, dry place away from sunlight to preserve their potency and prevent spoilage.

By following these guidelines, you'll use herbal remedies safely and effectively, harnessing nature's healing gifts responsibly.

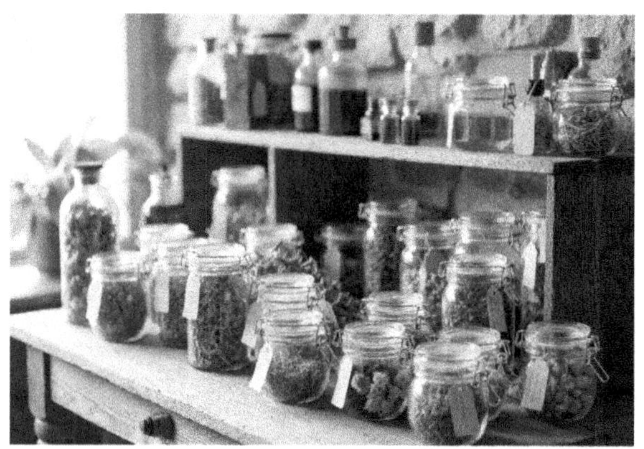

Foundations of Herbal Medicine

Understanding Herbal Traditions (African & Global)

Herbal medicine has been practiced across the world for millennia, with each culture developing unique approaches based on local flora and philosophies. African herbal traditions, for example, emphasize the spiritual connection between plants, people, and the environment. Many remedies are passed down orally and involve rituals, ceremonies, and deep respect for nature.

Similarly, traditional Chinese, Ayurvedic, Native American, and European herbal systems have rich histories and profound insights into healing. Despite cultural differences, common themes include using whole plants, balancing bodily systems, and treating the root cause rather than symptoms alone.

This book integrates knowledge from diverse traditions, focusing on plants accessible to many and remedies that have stood the test of time.

Plant Parts and Their Healing Properties

Different parts of a plant contain distinct chemical compounds, which determine their therapeutic effects:

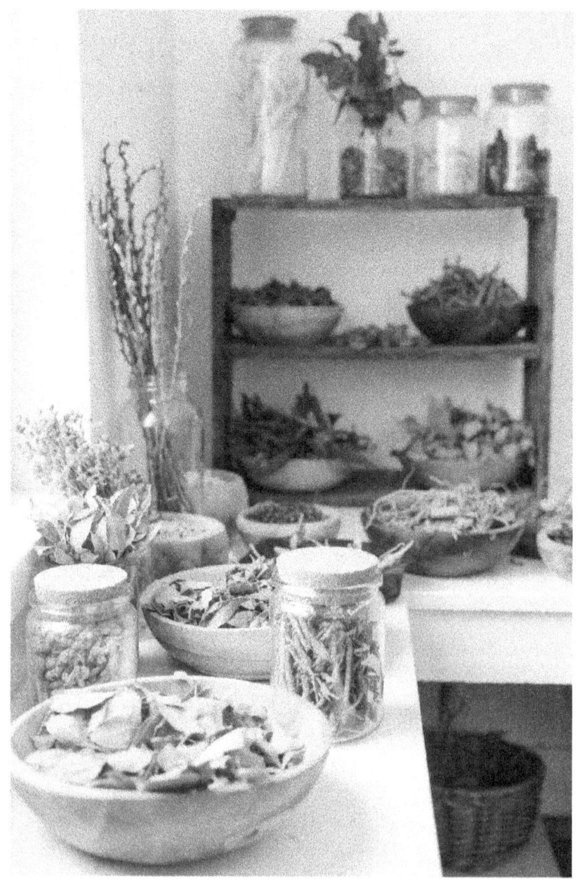

- **Roots and Rhizomes:** Often rich in concentrated compounds for long-term effects, such as anti-inflammatory or energizing properties.

- **Leaves:** Commonly used for teas and infusions, leaves usually contain volatile oils and antioxidants.

- **Barks and Stems:** Used for their astringent, antimicrobial, or circulatory benefits.

- **Flowers:** Typically fragrant and soothing, flowers are often used for mental health, relaxation, and skin treatments.

- **Seeds and Nuts:** Nutrient-dense and sometimes hormonal modulators.

- **Fruits and Peels:** Rich in vitamins, antioxidants, and immune-boosting compounds.

Understanding which part to use is critical for effectiveness and safety.

Preparation Methods Explained

The healing power of herbs depends on proper preparation. Common methods include:

- **Infusion:** Steeping leaves, flowers, or soft parts in hot water (like tea) to extract delicate compounds.

- **Decoction:** Boiling harder parts like roots or bark to release their active ingredients.

- **Tincture:** Extracting herbs in alcohol or vinegar for concentrated, longer-lasting preparations.

- **Poultice:** Applying crushed fresh or dried herbs directly on the skin to soothe inflammation or wounds.

- **Oil infusion:** Soaking herbs in oil to extract fat-soluble components for topical use.

Each method suits different plant parts and health goals. Detailed preparation instructions accompany every remedy in this book.

Dosage Principles & Measurement Guide

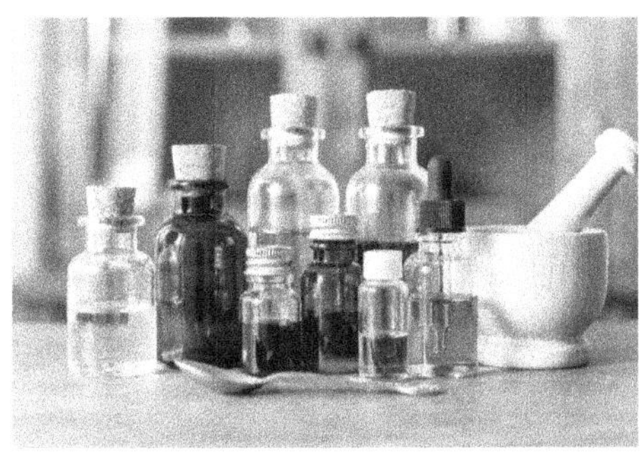

Proper dosing maximizes benefits while minimizing risks. Key points include:

- Use the smallest effective dose initially.

- Follow preparation-specific dosages (e.g., cups of tea, teaspoons of powder).

- Adjust doses carefully for children, elderly, or sensitive individuals.

- Avoid prolonged use unless recommended.

- Measure accurately using kitchen scales, spoons, or cups for consistency.

Conversion charts and dosage tables in the back matter assist with accurate measurement.

Safety, Toxicity, Interactions & Contraindications

Herbs are natural but not inherently safe for everyone. Some plants can cause side effects, allergic reactions, or interact negatively with medications.

- Always review caution notes for each remedy.

- Avoid herbs contraindicated in pregnancy, breastfeeding, or certain medical conditions.

- Be aware of potential allergies, especially if sensitive to related plants.

- Discontinue use immediately if adverse symptoms occur.

- Consult healthcare professionals before combining herbs with pharmaceuticals.

Safety awareness ensures herbal medicine is a supportive and empowering tool on your health journey.

SECTION I: ROOTS, RHIZOMES & TUBERS
(Remedies 1–60)

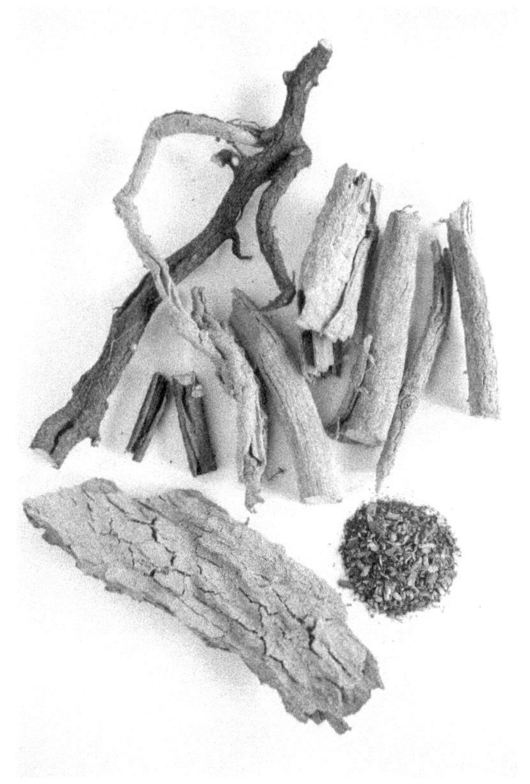

Digestive & Metabolic Roots :
Remedies 1–20

1. Ginger *(Zingiber officinale)*

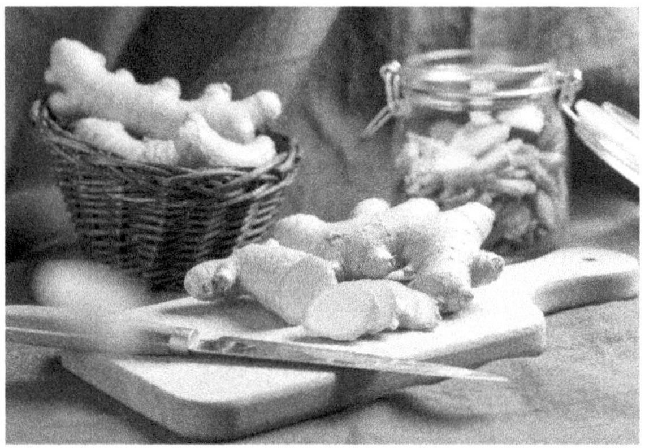

- *Part Used:* Rhizome

- *Traditional Uses:* Nausea, indigestion, cold, inflammation

- *Preparation:*

1. Wash a fresh ginger rhizome thoroughly.

2. Slice 5–7 thin pieces (about 1 tablespoon).

3. Add 1 1/2 cups of freshly boiled water.

4. Cover and steep for 10–15 minutes.

5. Strain and drink warm; honey may be added.

- *Dosage:* 1–2 cups daily

- *Caution:* Avoid excessive use with ulcers

2. Garlic (*Allium sativum*)

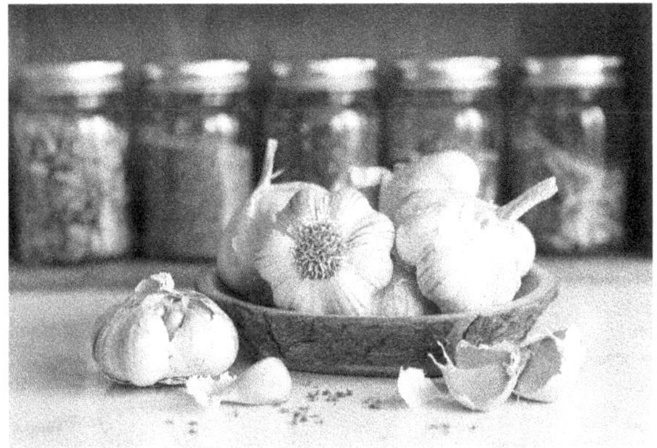

- *Part Used:* Bulb

- *Traditional Uses:* Hypertension, infections, immunity

- *Preparation:*

1. Peel and crush 1–2 fresh garlic cloves.

2. Allow to sit for 5 minutes to activate compounds.

3. Swallow with warm water or mix into food.

4. For tea, simmer crushed cloves in 1 cup of water for 5 minutes.

- *Dosage:* 1–2 cloves daily

- *Caution:* May increase bleeding risk

3. Turmeric (*Curcuma longa*)

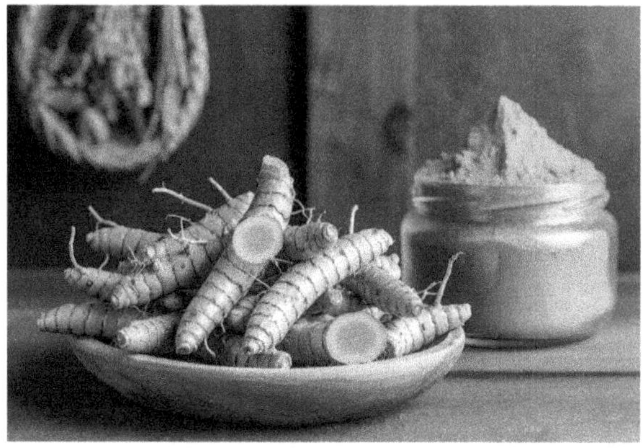

- *Part Used:* Rhizome

- *Traditional Uses:* Inflammation, joint pain, liver support

- *Preparation:*

1. Grate fresh turmeric or measure 1 teaspoon dried powder.

2. Add to 1 cup of water or milk.

3. Simmer gently for 5–10 minutes.

4. Add a pinch of black pepper before drinking.

- *Dosage:* 500–1000 mg daily

- *Caution:* Avoid with gallstones

4. Neem (*Azadirachta indica*)

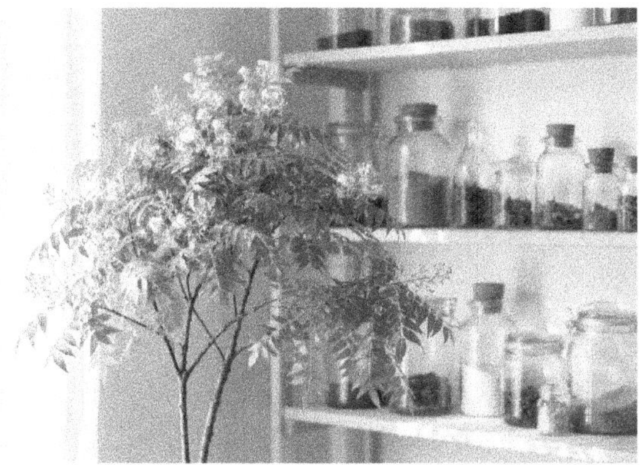

- ***Part Used:*** Leaves, bark

- ***Traditional Uses:*** Skin conditions, malaria support, detox

- ***Preparation:***

1. Wash a handful of fresh leaves (or 1 teaspoon dried).

2. Boil in 2 cups of water for 10–15 minutes.

3. Strain and allow to cool slightly before use.

- ***Dosage:*** Small cup once daily

- ***Caution:*** Not for pregnancy

5. Aloe Vera (*Aloe barbadensis*)

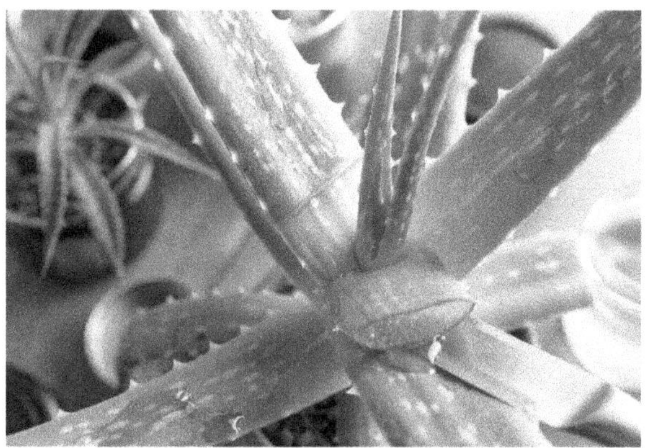

- *Part Used:* Gel

- *Traditional Uses:* Burns, constipation, skin hydration

- *Preparation:*

1. Cut a fresh aloe leaf and drain yellow latex.

2. Scoop out the clear gel.

3. Blend 1–2 tablespoons with water or juice.

- *Dosage:* 1–2 tablespoons

- *Caution:* Avoid long-term oral use

6. Bitter Leaf (*Vernonia amygdalina*)

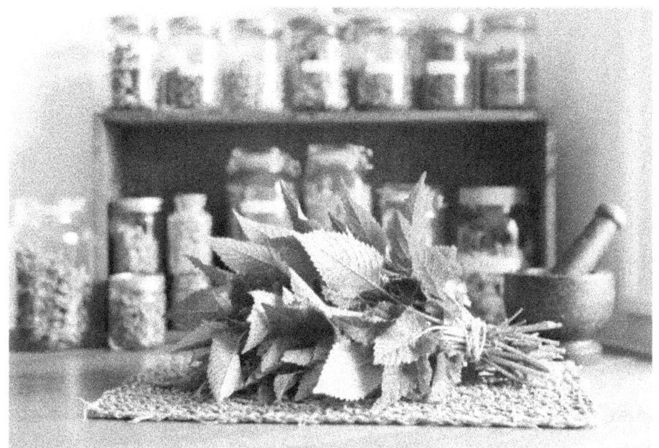

- *Part Used:* Leaves

- *Traditional Uses:* Diabetes support, digestion, malaria

- *Preparation:*

1. Wash fresh leaves thoroughly.

2. Squeeze and rinse repeatedly to reduce bitterness.

3. Boil lightly in water for 5–10 minutes.

4. Strain and drink.

- *Dosage:* ½ cup daily

- *Caution:* Bitter taste may cause nausea

7. Moringa (*Moringa oleifera*)

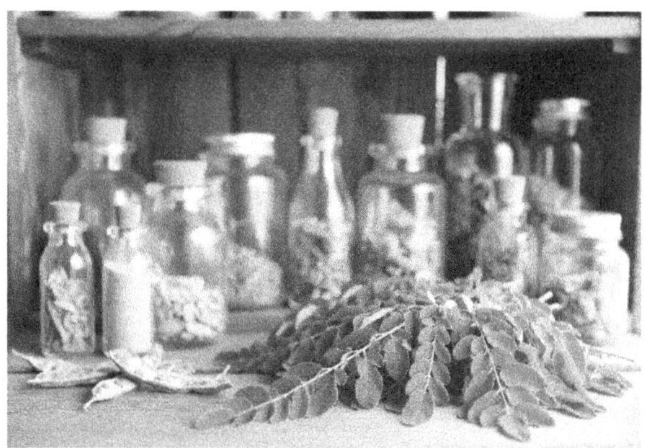

- *Part Used:* Leaves

- *Traditional Uses:* Nutrition, anemia, immunity

- *Preparation:*

1. Air-dry fresh leaves and grind into powder, or use fresh.

2. Add 1 teaspoon powder to warm water.

3. Stir well and drink.

- *Dosage:* 1–2 teaspoons daily

- *Caution:* Avoid root use

8. Lemongrass (*Cymbopogon citratus*)

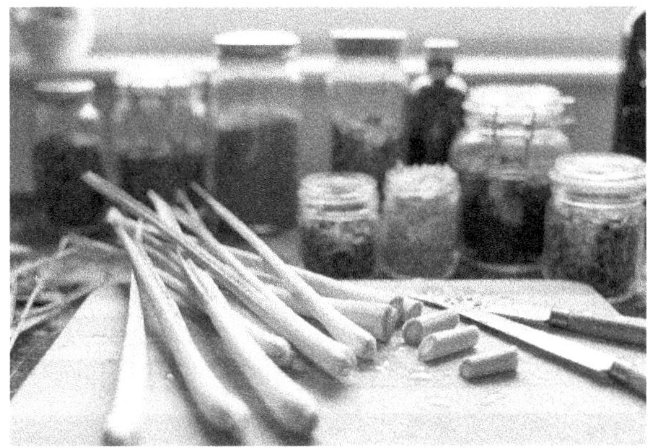

- *Part Used:* Leaves

- *Traditional Uses:* Fever, digestion, anxiety

- *Preparation:*

1. Wash and cut fresh stalks.

2. Crush lightly to release aroma.

3. Boil in 2 cups of water for 10 minutes.

4. Strain and drink warm.

- *Dosage:* 1–2 cups daily

- *Caution:* May lower blood pressure

9. Hibiscus (*Hibiscus sabdariffa*)

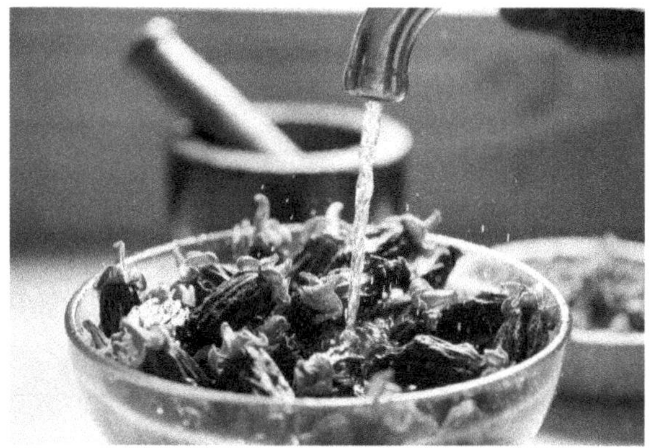

- *Part Used:* Calyces

- *Traditional Uses:* Hypertension, detox

- *Preparation:*

1. Rinse dried calyces thoroughly.

2. Add 1 tablespoon to 2 cups of hot water.

3. Steep for 10–15 minutes.

4. Strain and drink warm or chilled.

- *Dosage:* 1 cup daily

- *Caution:* Avoid with low BP

10. Clove (*Syzygium aromaticum*)

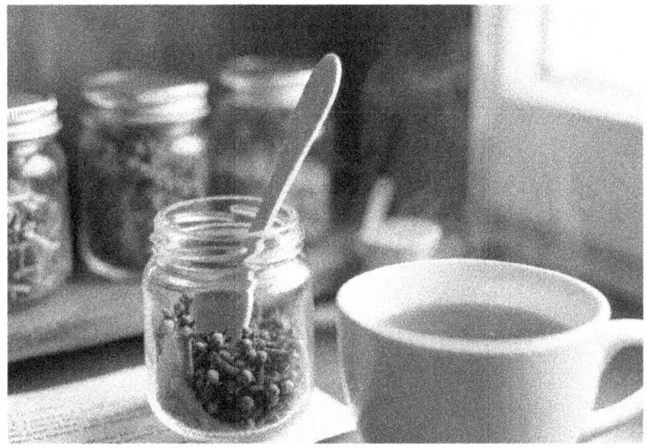

- *Part Used:* Flower buds

- *Traditional Uses:* Toothache, digestion

- *Preparation:*

1. Add 2–3 cloves to 1 cup of hot water.

2. Cover and steep for 10 minutes.

3. Strain and sip slowly or chew clove for tooth pain.

- *Dosage:* 1–2 cloves

- *Caution:* Excess may irritate mouth

11. Peppermint (*Mentha piperita*)

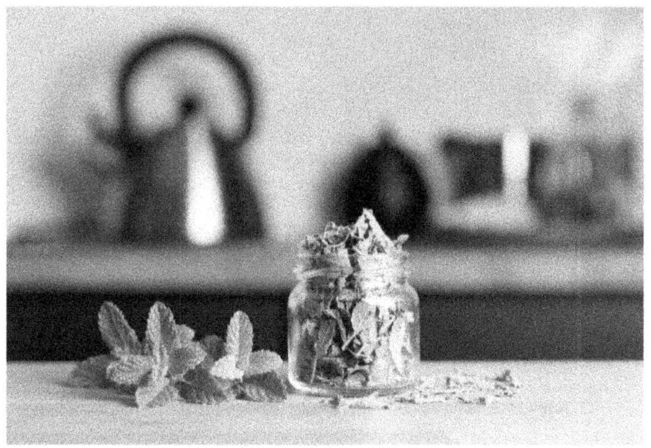

- ***Part Used:*** Leaves

- ***Traditional Uses:*** Bloating, headache

- ***Preparation:***

1. Add 1 tablespoon fresh or 1 teaspoon dried leaves to hot water.

2. Cover and steep for 10 minutes.

3. Strain before drinking.

- ***Dosage:*** 1–2 cups daily

- ***Caution:*** Avoid with GERD

12. Chamomile (*Matricaria chamomilla*)

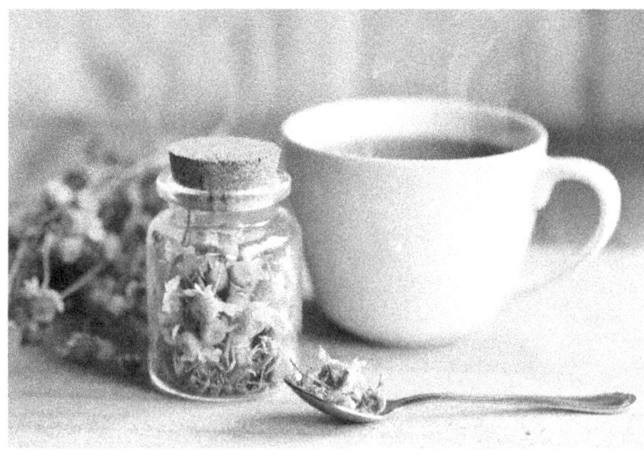

- *Part Used:* Flowers

- *Traditional Uses:* Sleep, anxiety

- *Preparation:*

1. Add 1 tablespoon dried flowers to hot water.

2. Cover and steep for 10 minutes.

3. Strain and drink before bedtime.

- *Dosage:* 1 cup at night

- *Caution:* Allergy to ragweed

13. Thyme (*Thymus vulgaris*)

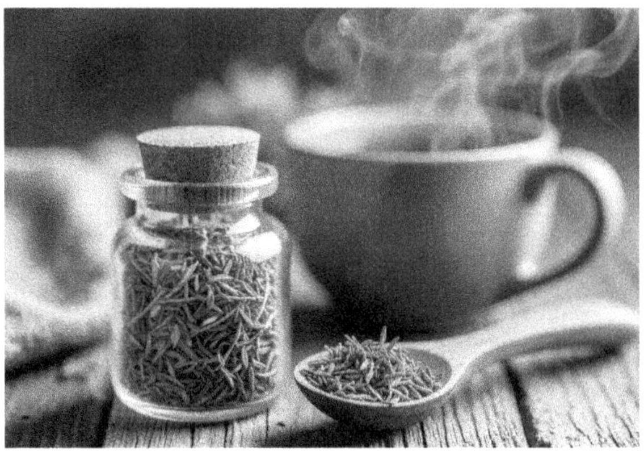

- *Part Used:* Leaves

- *Traditional Uses:* Cough, bronchitis

- *Preparation:*

1. Add 1 teaspoon dried thyme to hot water.

2. Steep for 10 minutes.

3. Strain and drink warm.

- *Dosage:* 1 cup daily

- *Caution:* Avoid excess in pregnancy

14. Scent Leaf (*Ocimum gratissimum*)

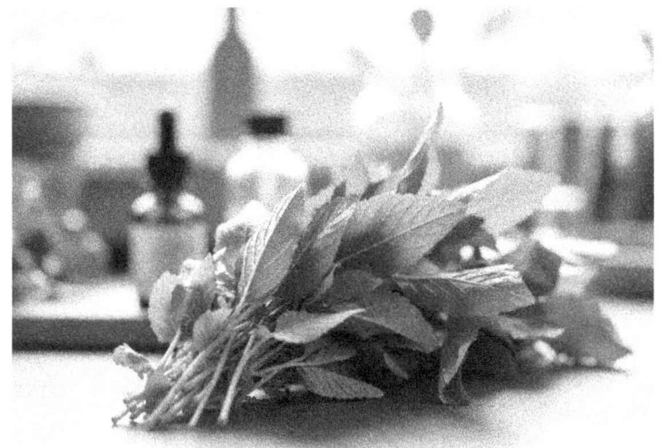

- ***Part Used:*** Leaves

- ***Traditional Uses:*** Diarrhea, cough, infections

- ***Preparation:***

1. Wash fresh leaves thoroughly.

2. Boil in 2 cups of water for 10 minutes.

3. Strain and drink warm.

- ***Dosage:*** ½–1 cup daily

- ***Caution:*** Strong aroma

15. Dandelion (*Taraxacum officinale*)

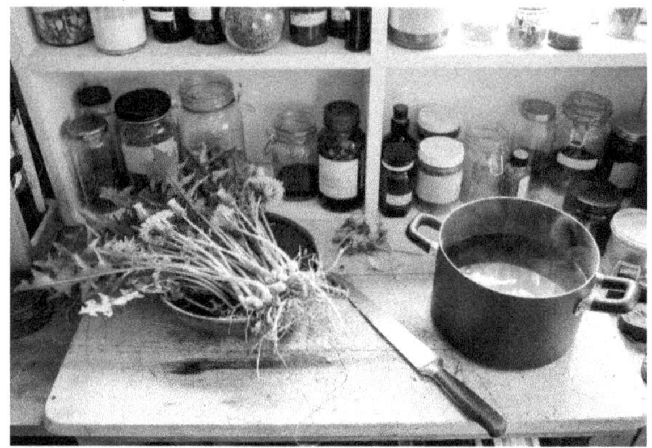

- *Part Used:* Leaves, root

- *Traditional Uses:* Liver support, diuretic

- *Preparation:*

1. Wash roots or leaves thoroughly.

2. Chop and boil in water for 10 minutes.

3. Strain and drink warm.

- *Dosage:* 1 cup daily

- *Caution:* Avoid bile obstruction

16. Cinnamon (*Cinnamomum verum*)

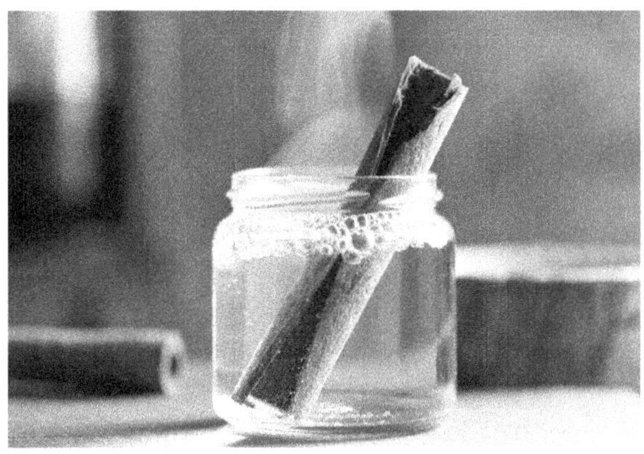

- *Part Used:* Bark

- *Traditional Uses:* Blood sugar support

- *Preparation:*

1. Break a small cinnamon stick.

2. Boil in 1½ cups of water for 10 minutes.

3. Strain and drink warm.

- *Dosage:* ½ teaspoon daily

- *Caution:* Avoid excess cassia

17. Eucalyptus (*Eucalyptus globulus*)

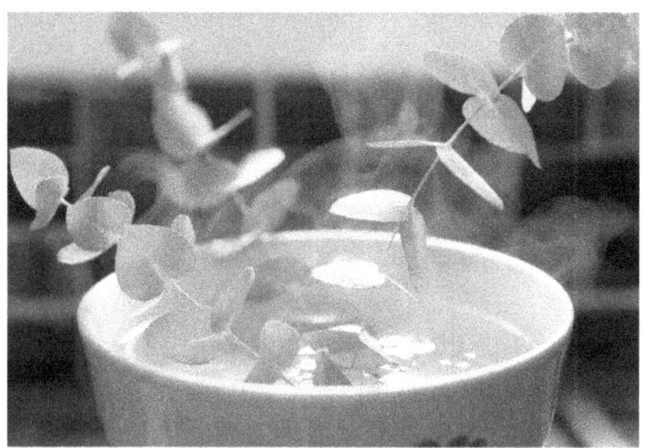

- *Part Used:* Leaves

- *Traditional Uses:* Cold, sinus congestion

- *Preparation:*

1. Add fresh leaves to a bowl of hot water.

2. Cover head with towel and inhale steam for 5–10 minutes.

- *Dosage:* As needed

- *Caution:* Not for children orally

18. Fennel (*Foeniculum vulgare*)

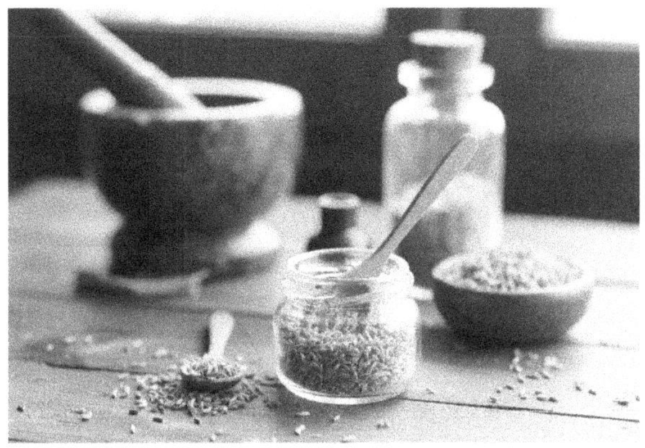

- *Part Used:* Seeds

- *Traditional Uses:* Gas, lactation support

- *Preparation:*

1. Lightly crush 1 teaspoon of seeds.

2. Add to hot water and steep for 10 minutes.

3. Strain before drinking.

- *Dosage:* 1 teaspoon seeds

- *Caution:* Avoid excess

19. Sage (*Salvia officinalis*)

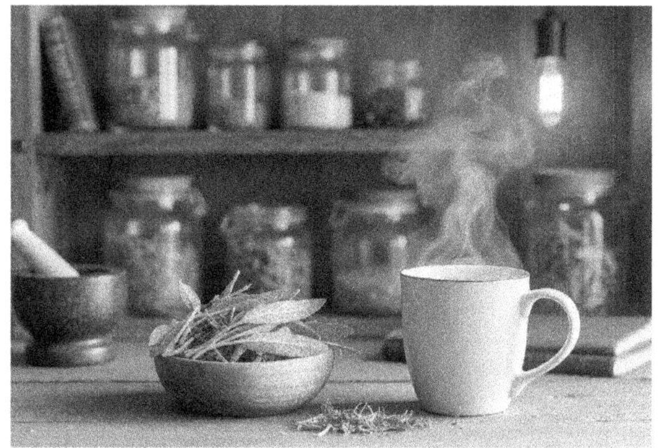

- *Part Used:* Leaves

- *Traditional Uses:* Sore throat, memory

- *Preparation:*

1. Add 1 teaspoon dried leaves to hot water.

2. Steep for 10 minutes.

3. Use as tea or gargle.

- *Dosage:* 1 cup daily

- *Caution:* Avoid prolonged use

20. Black Seed (*Nigella sativa*)

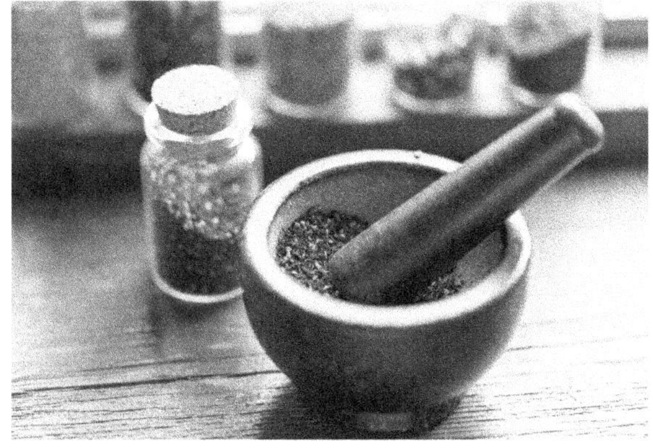

- *Part Used:* Seeds

- *Traditional Uses:* Immunity, asthma

- *Preparation:*

1. Lightly crush seeds using mortar.

2. Mix ½ teaspoon with honey or warm water.

3. Consume immediately.

- *Dosage:* ½ teaspoon daily

- *Caution:* Avoid pregnancy

Remedies 21–40
(Section I: Anti-inflammatory & Pain-relief Roots)

21. White Willow Bark (*Salix alba*)

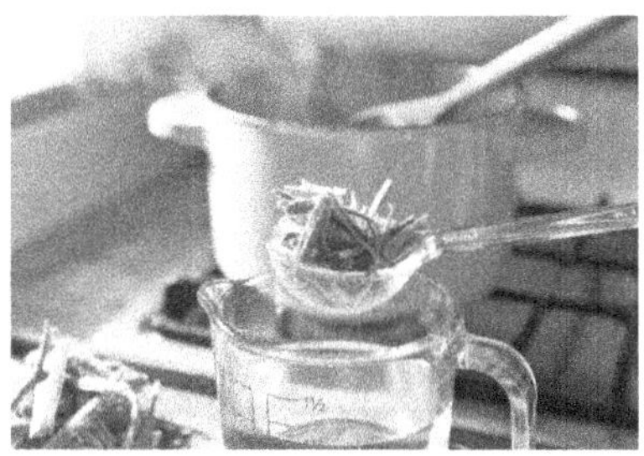

- *Part Used:* Bark

- *Traditional Uses:* Headache, back pain, arthritis, fever

- *Preparation:*

1. Measure 1 teaspoon of dried white willow bark.

2. Add to 1½ cups of cold water.

3. Bring to a gentle boil, then simmer for 10–15 minutes.

4. Strain and allow to cool slightly before drinking.

- *Dosage:* 1 cup once daily after meals

- *Caution:* Avoid if allergic to aspirin; not for children

22. Licorice Root (*Glycyrrhiza glabra*)

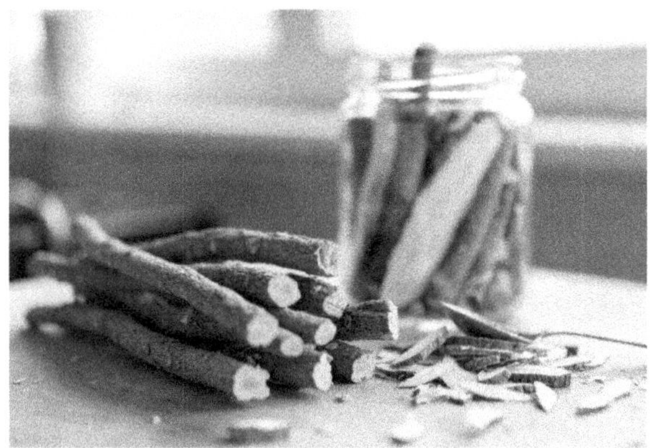

- *Part Used:* Root

- *Traditional Uses:* Ulcers, sore throat, cough, adrenal fatigue

- *Preparation:*

1. Crush or slice dried licorice root.

2. Add 1 teaspoon to 1½ cups of water.

3. Simmer gently for 10 minutes.

4. Strain and drink warm.

- *Dosage:* 1 cup daily for up to 2 weeks

- *Caution:* Avoid prolonged use if hypertensive

23. Ginseng (*Panax ginseng*)

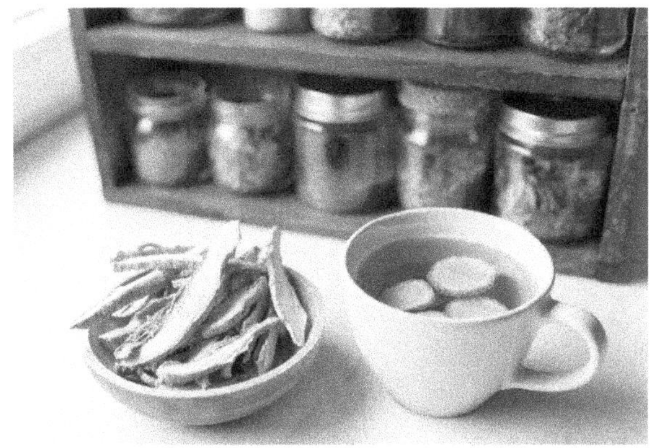

- *Part Used:* Root

- *Traditional Uses:* Fatigue, low immunity, poor stamina

- *Preparation:*

1. Slice dried ginseng root thinly.

2. Add 3–5 slices to hot (not boiling) water.

3. Cover and steep for 15 minutes.

4. Strain and drink.

- *Dosage:* 1 cup in the morning

- *Caution:* May cause insomnia if taken late

24. Ashwagandha (*Withania somnifera*)

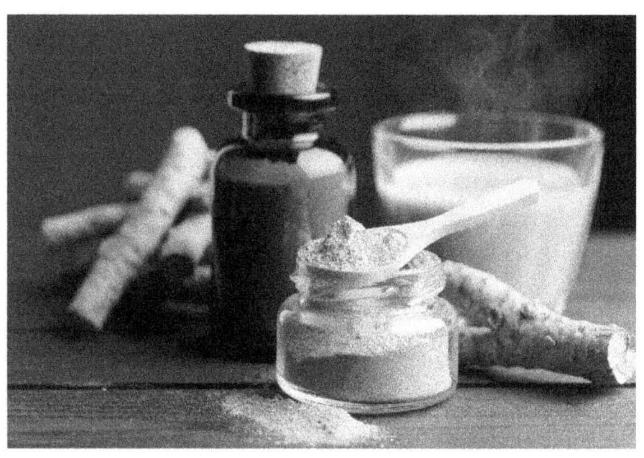

- *Part Used:* Root

- *Traditional Uses:* Stress, joint pain, nervous exhaustion

- *Preparation:*

1. Add 1 teaspoon of powdered root to a cup of warm water or milk.

2. Stir well until fully dissolved.

3. Drink slowly.

- *Dosage:* Once daily, preferably at night

- *Caution:* Avoid during pregnancy

25. Devil's Claw (*Harpagophytum procumbens*)

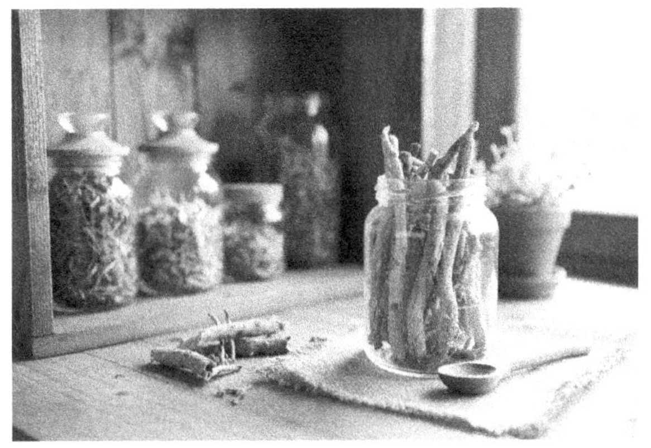

- *Part Used:* Root

- *Traditional Uses:* Arthritis, muscle and back pain

- *Preparation:*

1. Add 1 teaspoon of dried root to 2 cups of water.

2. Simmer for 15–20 minutes.

3. Strain and allow to cool.

- *Dosage:* ½ cup twice daily

- *Caution:* Avoid with stomach ulcers

26. Turmeric Root (*Curcuma longa*)

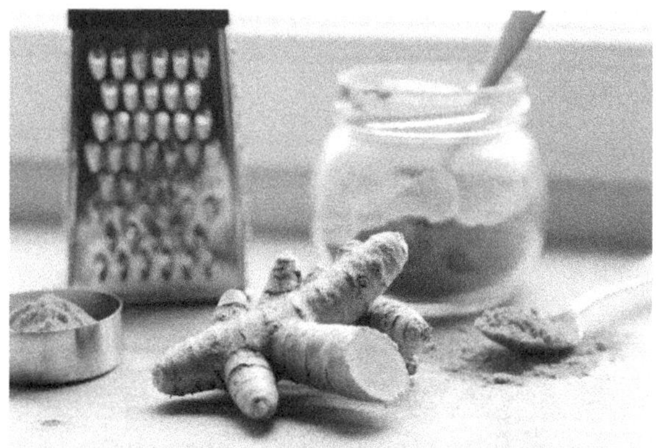

- *Part Used:* Rhizome

- *Traditional Uses:* Inflammation, joint pain, wound healing

- *Preparation:*

1. Grate fresh turmeric or measure 1 teaspoon of dried powder.

2. Add to a cup of water or milk.

3. Simmer for 5–10 minutes.

4. Add black pepper to enhance absorption.

- *Dosage:* 1 cup daily

- *Caution:* Avoid gallbladder disorders

27. Ginger Root (*Zingiber officinale*)

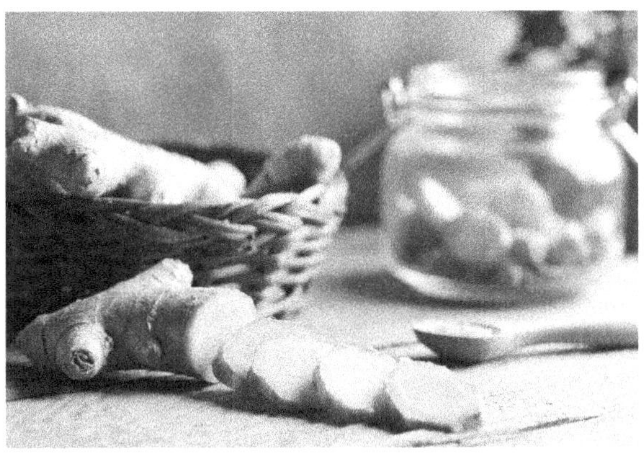

- *Part Used:* Rhizome

- *Traditional Uses:* Muscle pain, nausea, poor circulation

- *Preparation:*

1. Slice 5–6 pieces of fresh ginger.

2. Add to 1½ cups of boiling water.

3. Steep for 10 minutes.

4. Strain and drink warm.

- *Dosage:* 1–2 cups daily

- *Caution:* Avoid excess with ulcers

28. Burdock Root (*Arctium lappa*)

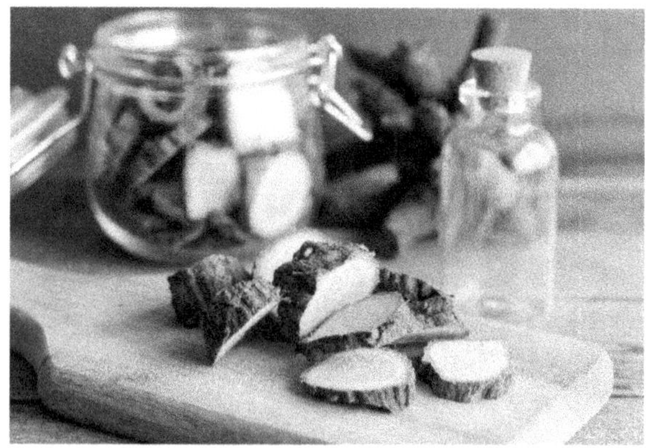

- *Part Used:* Root

- *Traditional Uses:* Blood cleansing, eczema, joint pain

- *Preparation:*

1. Chop dried burdock root.

2. Add 1 tablespoon to 2 cups of water.

3. Simmer for 15 minutes.

4. Strain before use.

- *Dosage:* 1 cup daily

- *Caution:* May cause frequent urination

29. Yellow Dock (*Rumex crispus*)

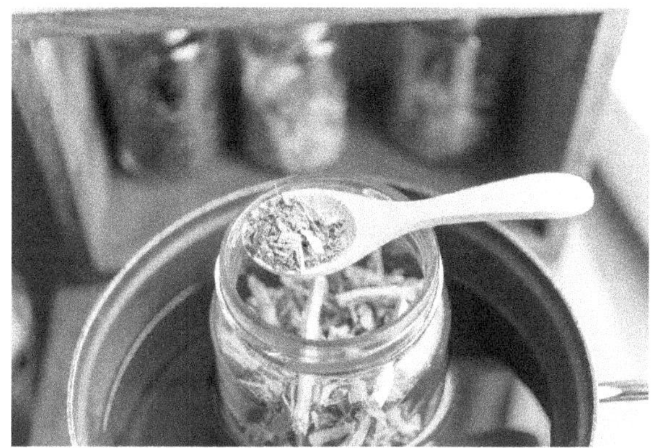

- *Part Used:* Root

- *Traditional Uses:* Constipation, iron deficiency support

- *Preparation:*

1. Add ½–1 teaspoon of dried root to 1½ cups of water.

2. Simmer gently for 10 minutes.

3. Strain and drink warm.

- *Dosage:* Small cup once daily

- *Caution:* Avoid diarrhea

30. Kava Kava (*Piper methysticum*)

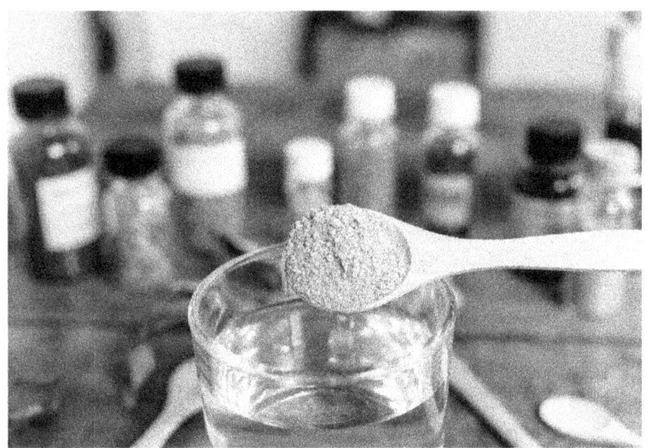

- ***Part Used:*** Root

- ***Traditional Uses:*** Anxiety, muscle tension, pain

- ***Preparation:***

1. Place 1 teaspoon of powdered root in warm (not hot) water.

2. Knead or stir for several minutes.

3. Strain before drinking.

- ***Dosage:*** Short-term use only

- ***Caution:*** Risk of liver toxicity

31. African Ginger (*Siphonochilus aethiopicus*)

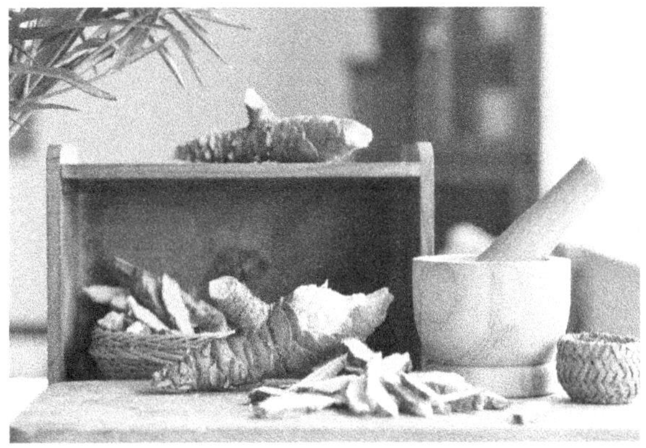

- *Part Used:* Rhizome

- *Traditional Uses:* Pain, asthma, respiratory infections

- *Preparation:*

1. Crush fresh rhizome or use dried slices.

2. Boil in 1½ cups of water for 10 minutes.

3. Strain and drink warm.

- *Dosage:* 1 cup daily

- *Caution:* Avoid pregnancy

32. Valerian Root (*Valeriana officinalis*)

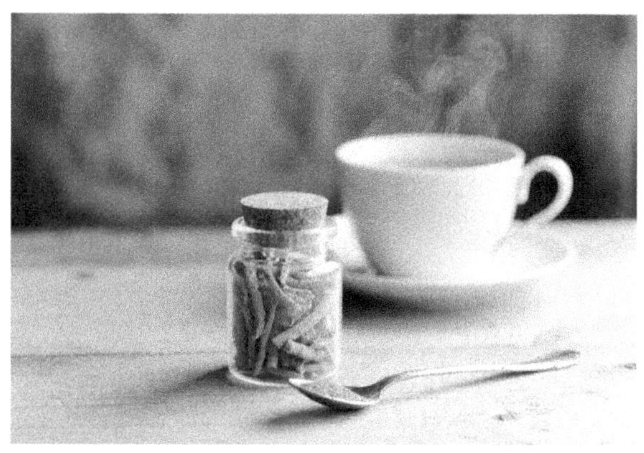

- *Part Used:* Root

- *Traditional Uses:* Muscle pain, insomnia, anxiety

- *Preparation:*

1. Add 1 teaspoon of dried root to hot water.

2. Cover and steep for 10–15 minutes.

3. Strain before use.

- *Dosage:* 1 cup at night

- *Caution:* Causes drowsiness

33. Maca Root (*Lepidium meyenii*)

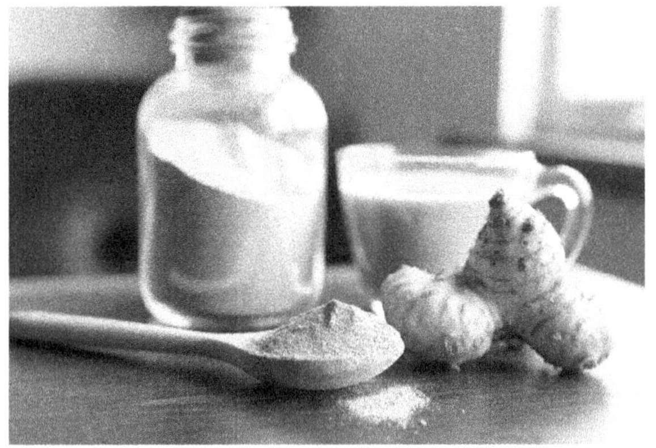

- *Part Used:* Root

- *Traditional Uses:* Energy, fertility, hormonal balance

- *Preparation:*

1. Add 1 teaspoon of maca powder to warm water or smoothies.

2. Stir until fully mixed.

- *Dosage:* Once daily

- *Caution:* Avoid with thyroid disorders

34. Kudzu Root (*Pueraria lobata*)

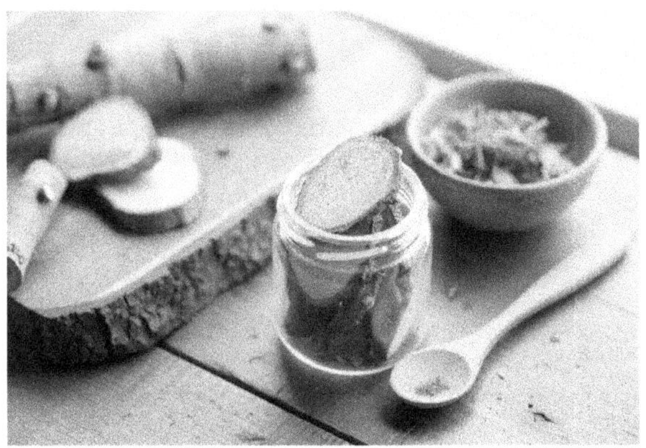

- *Part Used:* Root

- *Traditional Uses:* Muscle pain, alcohol dependence support

- *Preparation:*

1. Slice dried root thinly.

2. Boil in 2 cups of water for 15 minutes.

3. Strain before drinking.

- *Dosage:* 1 cup daily

- *Caution:* Hormonal sensitivity

35. Angelica (*Angelica archangelica*)

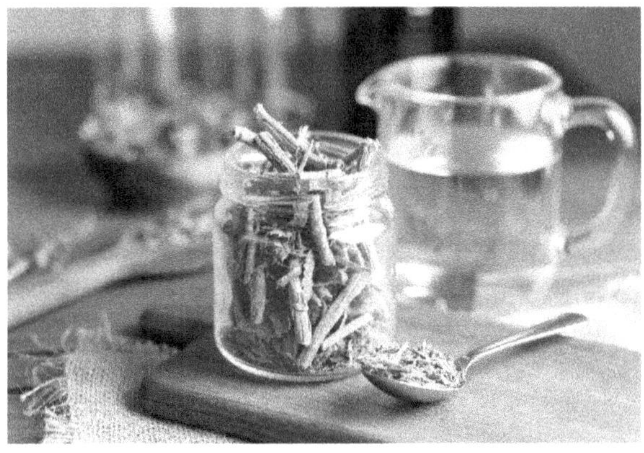

- *Part Used:* Root

- *Traditional Uses:* Joint pain, circulation, cramps

- *Preparation:*

1. Add 1 teaspoon of dried root to 1½ cups of water.

2. Simmer for 10 minutes.

3. Strain and drink warm.

- *Dosage:* 1 cup daily

- *Caution:* Photosensitivity

36. Sarsaparilla (*Smilax officinalis*)

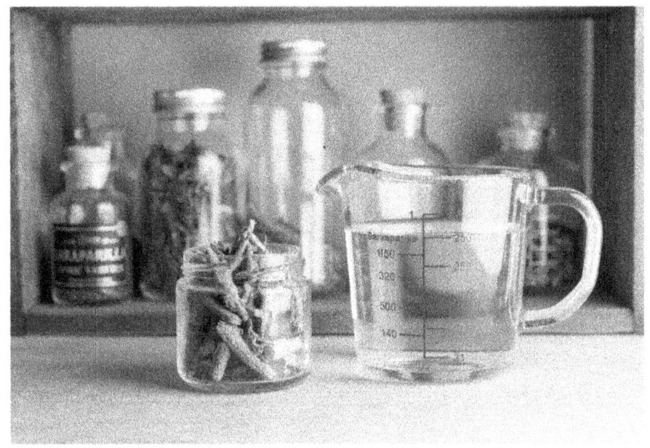

- *Part Used:* Root

- *Traditional Uses:* Arthritis, skin disorders

- *Preparation:*

1. Add 1 tablespoon of dried root to 2 cups of water.

2. Simmer for 15 minutes.

3. Strain before use.

- *Dosage:* 1 cup daily

- *Caution:* Avoid excessive use

37. Peony Root (*Paeonia lactiflora*)

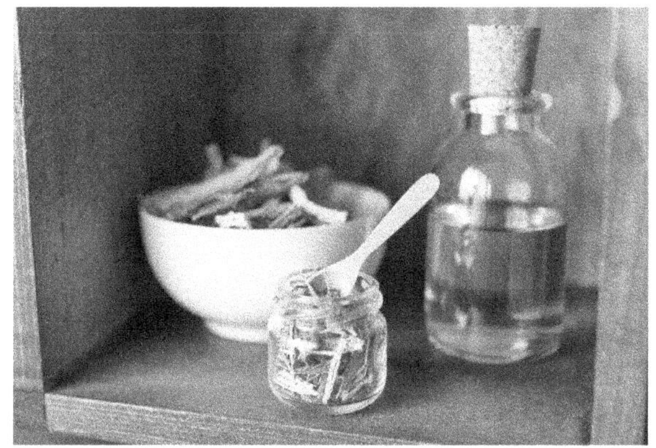

- *Part Used:* Root

- *Traditional Uses:* Muscle cramps, inflammation

- *Preparation:*

1. Add 1 teaspoon of dried root to water.

2. Simmer for 10 minutes.

3. Strain before drinking.

- *Dosage:* Small cup daily

- *Caution:* Avoid pregnancy

38. Goldenseal (*Hydrastis canadensis*)

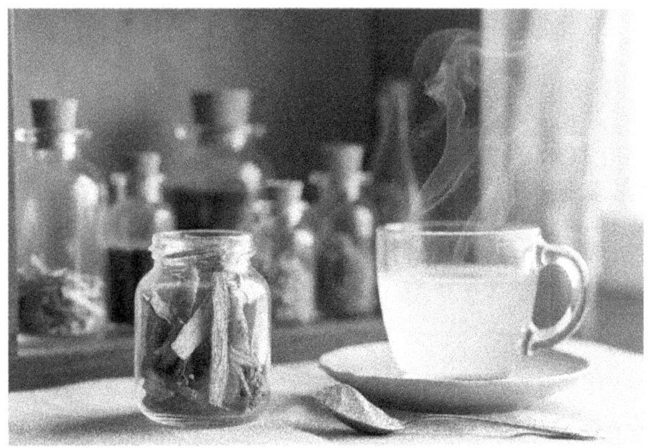

- ***Part Used:*** Root

- ***Traditional Uses:*** Infections, inflammation

- ***Preparation:***

1. Add ½ teaspoon of powdered root to hot water.

2. Steep for 10 minutes.

3. Strain and drink.

- ***Dosage:*** Short-term use only

- ***Caution:*** Avoid long-term use

39. Yarrow Root (*Achillea millefolium*)

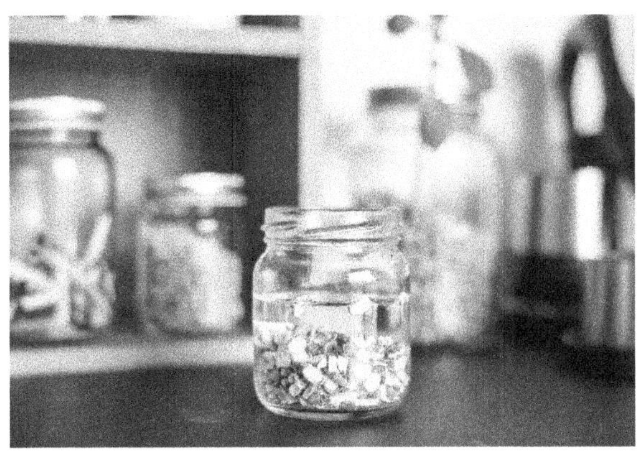

- *Part Used:* Root

- *Traditional Uses:* Pain, wound healing

- *Preparation:*

1. Add 1 teaspoon of chopped root to water.

2. Simmer for 10 minutes.

3. Strain before use.

- *Dosage:* 1 cup daily

- *Caution:* Allergy risk

40. Solomon's Seal (*Polygonatum odoratum*)

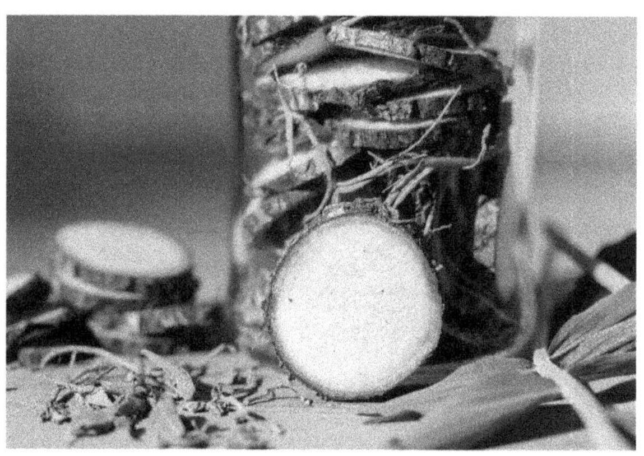

- *Part Used:* Root

- *Traditional Uses:* Joint lubrication, tendon and ligament pain

- *Preparation:*

1. Slice dried root thinly.

2. Simmer in 2 cups of water for 20 minutes.

3. Strain and allow to cool slightly.

- *Dosage:* 1 cup daily

- *Caution:* Proper identification is essential

Immune-boosting & Fever-support Roots (41-60)

41. Echinacea (*Echinacea purpurea*)

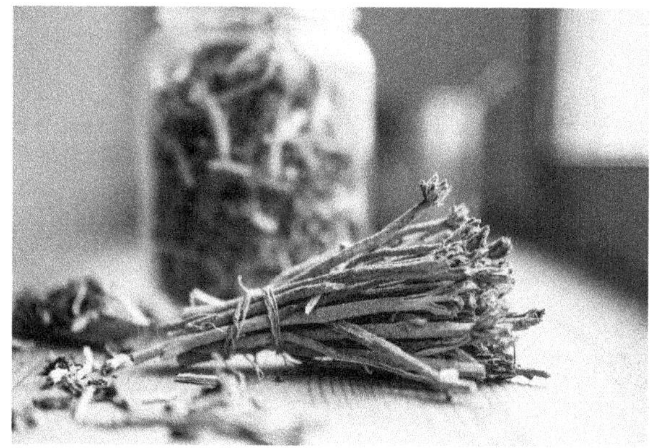

- *Part Used:* Root

- *Traditional Uses:* Immunity support, cold, flu, infections

- *Preparation:*

1. Chop dried echinacea root.

2. Add 1 teaspoon to 1½ cups of water.

3. Simmer gently for 10–15 minutes.

4. Strain and drink warm.

- *Dosage:* 1 cup once daily for 7–10 days

- *Caution:* Avoid long-term continuous use

42. Baobab Root (*Adansonia digitata*)

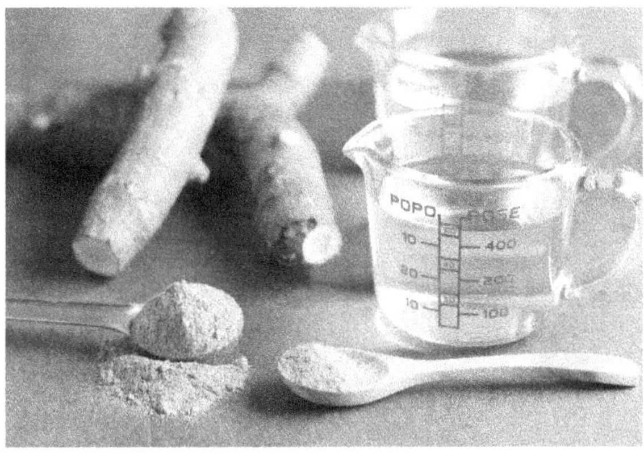

- *Part Used:* Root bark

- *Traditional Uses:* Fever, immune weakness, digestive support

- *Preparation:*

1. Rinse dried root bark thoroughly.

2. Add 1 tablespoon to 2 cups of water.

3. Boil for 15 minutes.

4. Strain and drink.

- *Dosage:* 1 cup daily

- *Caution:* Use moderate amounts

43. Astragalus (*Astragalus membranaceus*)

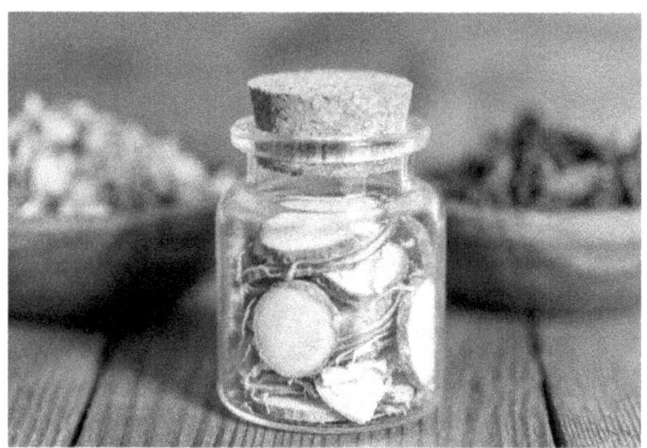

- ***Part Used:*** Root

- ***Traditional Uses:*** Immune tonic, fatigue, frequent illness

- ***Preparation:***

1. Slice dried root thinly.

2. Add 3–4 slices to 2 cups of water.

3. Simmer for 20 minutes.

4. Strain before use.

- ***Dosage:*** 1 cup daily

- ***Caution:*** Avoid during acute fever

44. African Wild Potato (*Hypoxis hemerocallidea*)

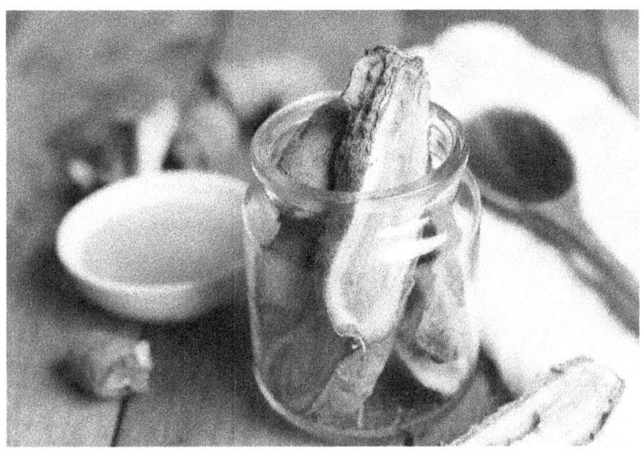

- *Part Used:* Tuber

- *Traditional Uses:* Immune support, inflammation, infections

- *Preparation:*

1. Wash and slice dried tuber.

2. Boil 1 teaspoon in 2 cups of water for 15 minutes.

3. Strain and allow to cool slightly.

- *Dosage:* ½–1 cup daily

- *Caution:* Avoid excessive use

45. Fever Root (*Caesalpinia bonduc*)

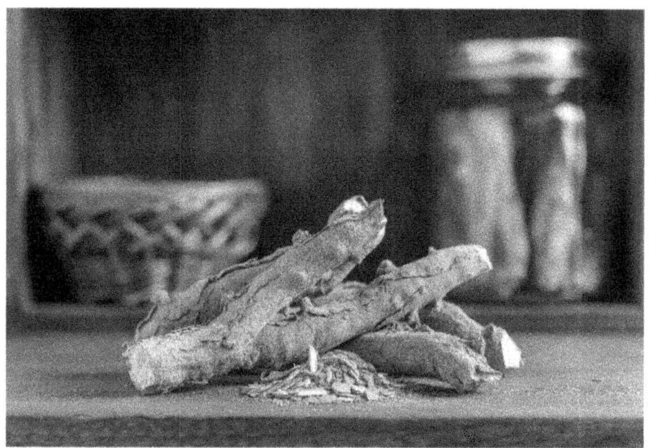

- ***Part Used:*** Root

- ***Traditional Uses:*** Fever, malaria support, chills

- ***Preparation:***

1. Crush dried root lightly.

2. Add 1 tablespoon to 2 cups of water.

3. Boil for 15–20 minutes.

4. Strain before drinking.

- ***Dosage:*** ½ cup twice daily

- ***Caution:*** Very bitter; avoid overdose

46. Elecampane (*Inula helenium*)

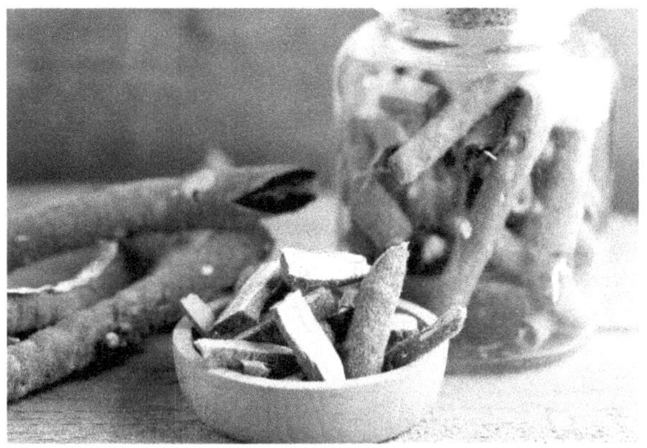

- *Part Used:* Root

- *Traditional Uses:* Cough, bronchial infections, immunity

- *Preparation:*

1. Chop dried root.

2. Add 1 teaspoon to 1½ cups of water.

3. Simmer for 10–15 minutes.

4. Strain and drink warm.

- *Dosage:* 1 cup daily

- *Caution:* Avoid pregnancy

47. Goldthread (*Coptis chinensis*)

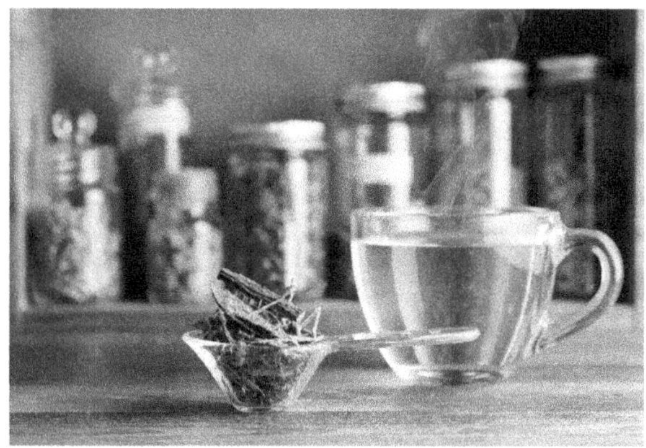

- ***Part Used:*** Rhizome

- ***Traditional Uses:*** Fever, infections, digestive infections

- ***Preparation:***

1. Add ½ teaspoon dried rhizome to hot water.

2. Cover and steep for 10 minutes.

3. Strain before drinking.

- ***Dosage:*** Small cup once daily

- ***Caution:*** Avoid long-term use

48. Pellitory Root (*Anacyclus pyrethrum*)

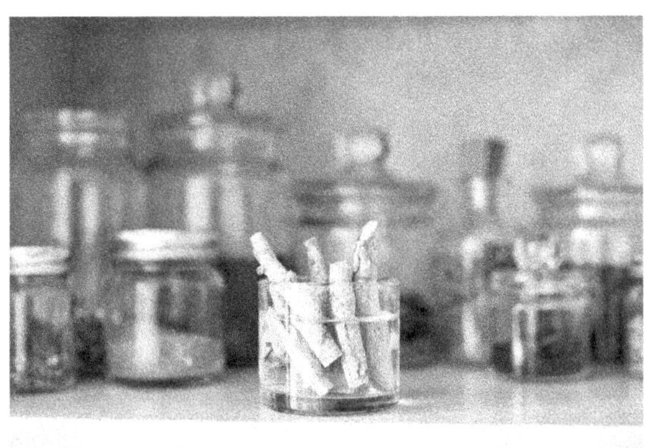

- *Part Used:* Root

- *Traditional Uses:* Fever, toothache, immune stimulation

- *Preparation:*

1. Add ½ teaspoon dried root to water.

2. Boil gently for 10 minutes.

3. Strain and drink warm.

- *Dosage:* Small cup daily

- *Caution:* Strong taste; use sparingly

49. Yellow Gentian (*Gentiana lutea*)

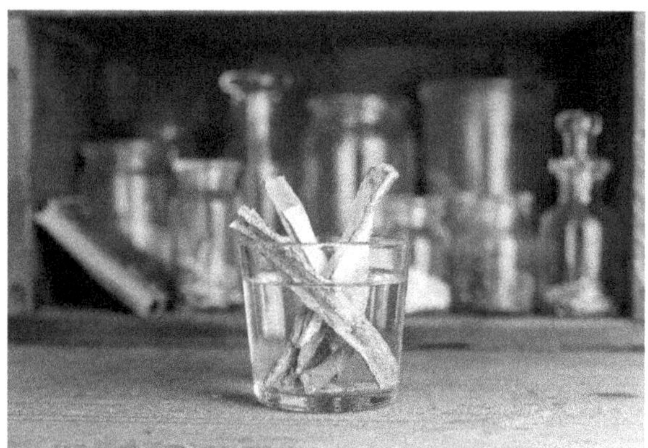

- ***Part Used:*** Root

- ***Traditional Uses:*** Fever, digestive weakness, appetite loss

- ***Preparation:***

1. Add ½ teaspoon dried root to cold water.

2. Soak for 8–12 hours (cold infusion).

3. Strain before use.

- ***Dosage:*** Small cup once daily

- ***Caution:*** Avoid ulcers

50. Sweet Flag (*Acorus calamus*)

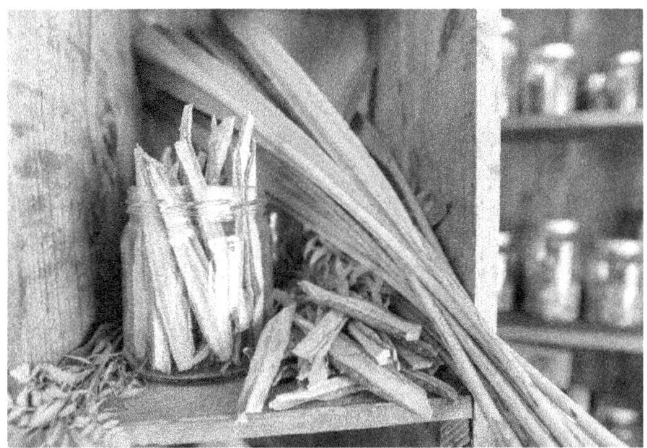

- ***Part Used:*** Rhizome

- ***Traditional Uses:*** Fever, digestive disorders, infections

- ***Preparation:***

1. Slice dried rhizome.

2. Add 1 teaspoon to 1½ cups of water.

3. Simmer for 10 minutes.

4. Strain before drinking.

- ***Dosage:*** ½–1 cup daily

- ***Caution:*** Use only small doses

51. Oregon Grape Root (*Mahonia aquifolium*)

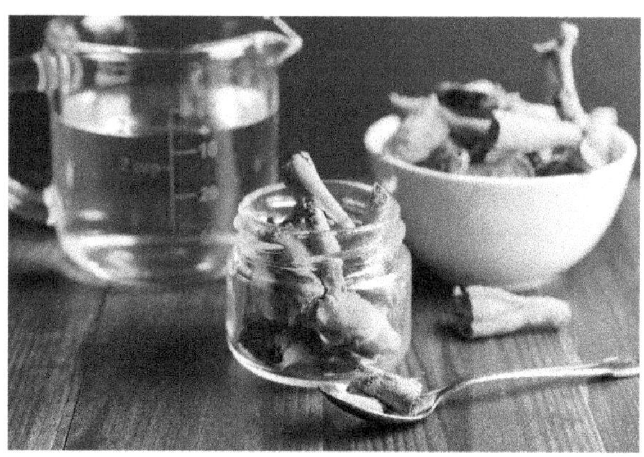

- *Part Used:* Root

- **Traditional Uses:** Infections, liver support, immunity

- *Preparation:*

1. Add 1 teaspoon dried root to 2 cups of water.

2. Simmer for 15 minutes.

3. Strain before use.

- *Dosage:* 1 cup daily

- *Caution:* Avoid pregnancy

52. Poke Root (*Phytolacca americana*)

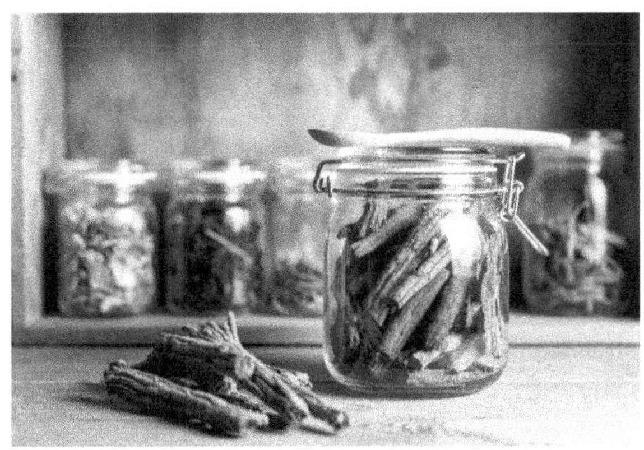

- *Part Used:* Root

- *Traditional Uses:* Immune stimulation, swollen glands

- *Preparation:*

1. Use only professionally dried root.

2. Add a *pinch* to 2 cups of water.

3. Simmer for 10 minutes.

4. Strain thoroughly.

- *Dosage:* Very small amounts only

- *Caution:* Toxic in excess; expert supervision advised

53. African Licorice (*Abrus precatorius*)

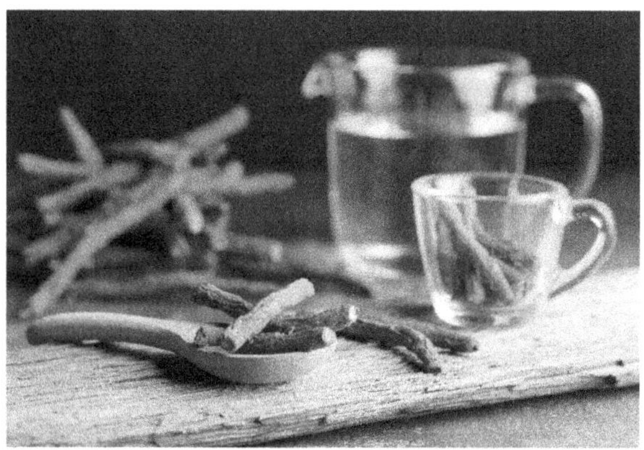

- *Part Used:* Root (NOT seeds)

- *Traditional Uses:* Fever, cough, throat infections

- *Preparation:*

1. Use properly identified dried root only.

2. Add ½ teaspoon to 2 cups of water.

3. Boil for 10 minutes.

4. Strain before drinking.

- *Dosage:* Small cup once daily

- *Caution:* Seeds are toxic; root only

54. Marshmallow Root (*Althaea officinalis*)

- ***Part Used:*** Root

- ***Traditional Uses:*** Fever, sore throat, inflammation

- ***Preparation:***

1. Add 1 tablespoon chopped root to cold water.

2. Soak for 4–6 hours.

3. Strain and drink.

- ***Dosage:*** 1 cup daily

- ***Caution:*** May delay absorption of medications

55. Gentianella (*Gentianella alborosea*)

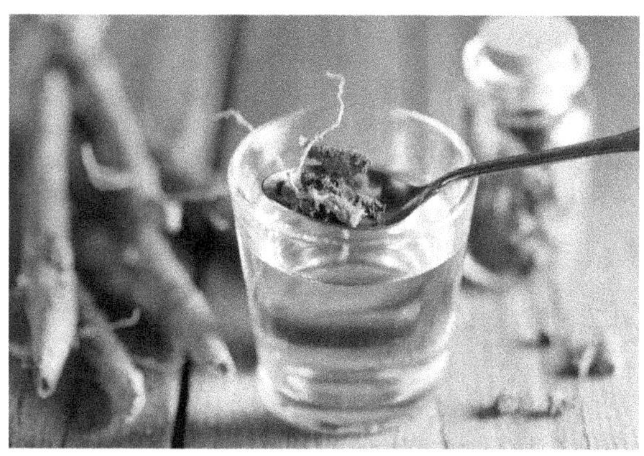

- *Part Used:* Root

- *Traditional Uses:* Fever, infections, digestive weakness

- *Preparation:*

1. Add ½ teaspoon dried root to water.

2. Simmer for 10 minutes.

3. Strain before use.

- *Dosage:* Small cup daily

- *Caution:* Avoid pregnancy

56. Calumba Root (*Jateorhiza palmata*)

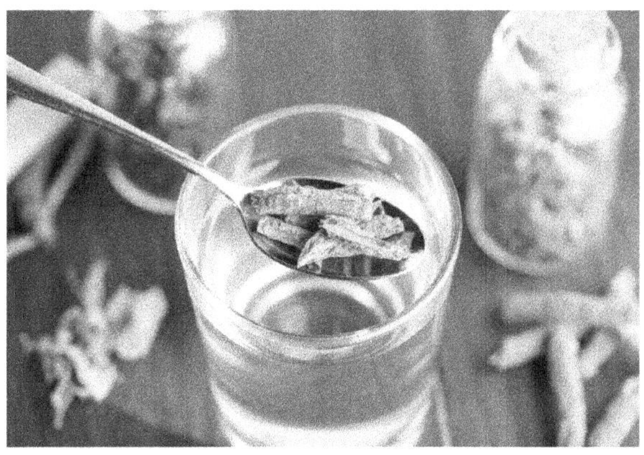

- *Part Used:* Root

- *Traditional Uses:* Fever, digestive infections

- *Preparation:*

1. Add ½ teaspoon dried root to water.

2. Steep in hot water for 10 minutes.

3. Strain before drinking.

- *Dosage:* Small cup daily

- *Caution:* Avoid ulcers

57. Snake Root (*Rauvolfia serpentina*)

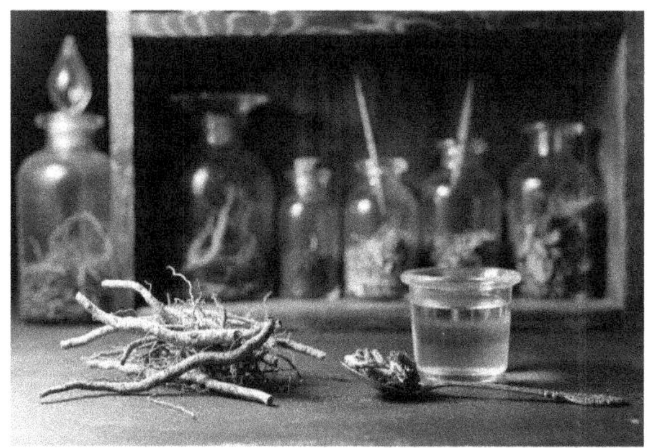

- *Part Used:* Root

- *Traditional Uses:* Fever, hypertension, nervous disorders

- *Preparation:*

1. Add ½ teaspoon dried root to water.

2. Simmer for 10 minutes.

3. Strain and drink.

- *Dosage:* Small cup daily

- *Caution:* Avoid with depression

58. Wild Indigo (*Baptisia tinctoria*)

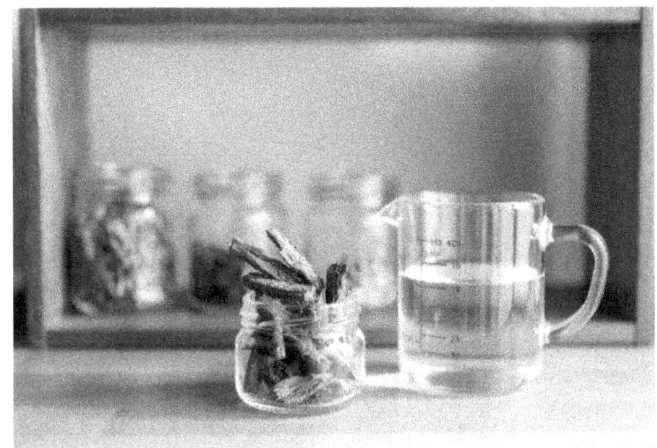

- *Part Used:* Root

- *Traditional Uses:* Fever, infections, immune stimulation

- *Preparation:*

1. Add ½ teaspoon dried root to 2 cups of water.

2. Simmer for 10 minutes.

3. Strain before use.

- *Dosage:* Small cup daily

- *Caution:* Use short-term only

59. Japanese Knotweed (*Polygonum cuspidatum*)

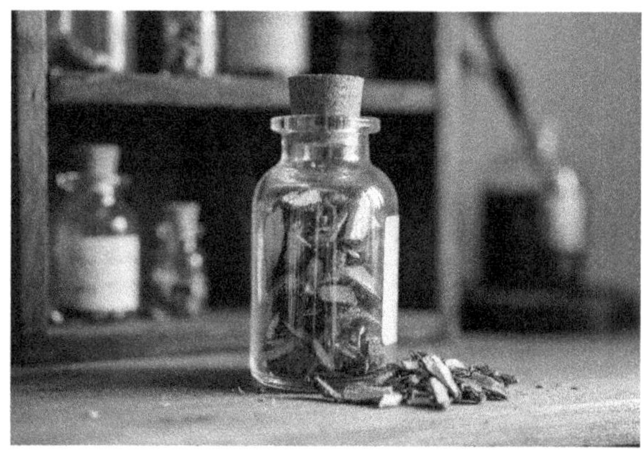

- *Part Used:* Root

- *Traditional Uses:* Fever, inflammation, immune support

- *Preparation:*

1. Chop dried root.

2. Add 1 teaspoon to 1½ cups of water.

3. Simmer for 15 minutes.

4. Strain and drink.

- *Dosage:* 1 cup daily

- *Caution:* Avoid pregnancy

60. Neem Root (*Azadirachta indica*)

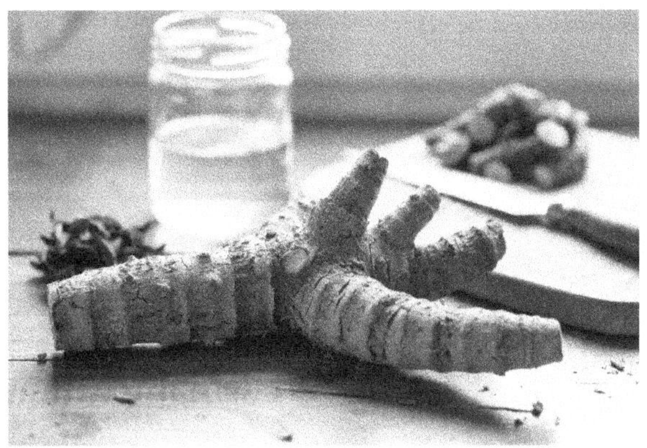

- *Part Used:* Root

- *Traditional Uses:* Fever, infections, immune cleansing

- *Preparation:*

1. Wash and chop dried neem root.

2. Boil 1 teaspoon in 2 cups of water for 15 minutes.

3. Strain and allow to cool.

- *Dosage:* ½–1 cup daily

- *Caution:* Avoid prolonged use

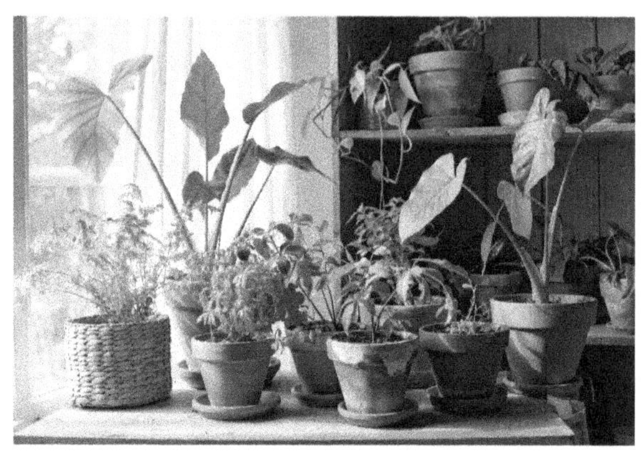

SECTION II: LEAVES & GREEN HERBS
(Remedies 61–140)

Blood Tonic & Anemia-support
Leaves (61–80)

61. Neem (*Azadirachta indica*)

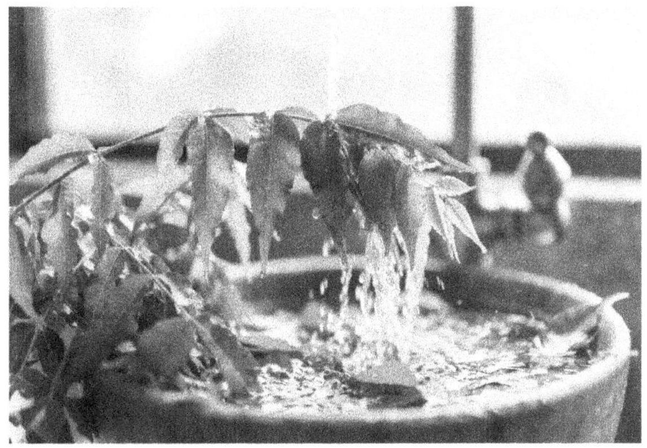

- ***Part Used:*** Leaves

- ***Traditional Uses:*** Blood purification, infections

- ***Preparation:*** Wash fresh leaves thoroughly. Boil 1 tablespoon of chopped leaves in 2 cups of water for 15 minutes. Strain and allow to cool.

- ***Dosage:*** ½ cup once daily for up to 7 days

- ***Caution:*** Avoid in pregnancy; do not use long-term

62. Bitter Leaf (*Vernonia amygdalina*)

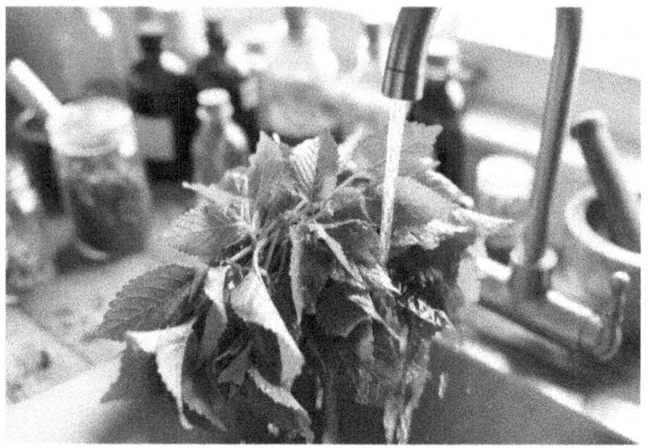

- *Part Used:* Leaves

- *Traditional Uses:* Blood sugar control, digestion

- *Preparation:* Wash leaves and squeeze repeatedly to reduce bitterness. Boil a handful in 3 cups of water for 10 minutes. Strain.

- *Dosage:* 1 cup daily

- *Caution:* Excess may cause nausea

63. Moringa (*Moringa oleifera*)

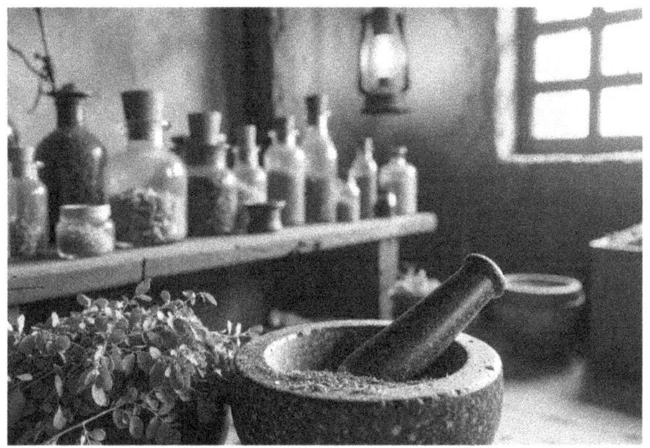

- ***Part Used:*** Leaves

- ***Traditional Uses:*** Nutrition, anemia, metabolism

- ***Preparation:*** Air-dry leaves, grind into powder. Steep 1 teaspoon in hot water for 5 minutes.

- ***Dosage:*** 1 cup daily or 1 teaspoon powder in meals

- ***Caution:*** Avoid excessive use

64. Mint (*Mentha piperita*)

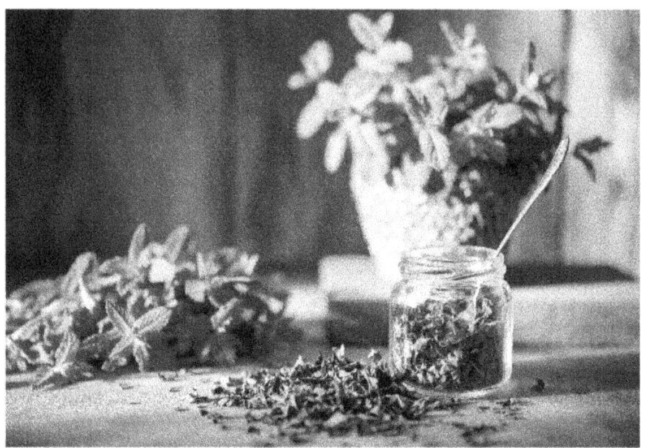

- *Part Used:* Leaves

- *Traditional Uses:* Indigestion, bloating

- *Preparation:* Crush fresh leaves. Pour boiling water over 1 tablespoon and steep for 5–7 minutes.

- *Dosage:* After meals

- *Caution:* Avoid reflux sensitivity

65. Basil (*Ocimum gratissimum*)

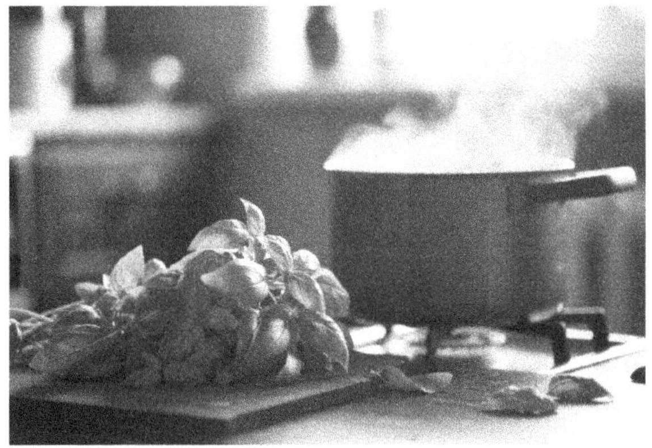

- *Part Used:* Leaves

- *Traditional Uses:* Gas, mild infections

- *Preparation:* Wash and boil a handful of leaves in 2 cups of water for 10 minutes. Strain.

- *Dosage:* 1 cup daily

- *Caution:* Safe in moderation

66. Scent Leaf (*Ocimum viride*)

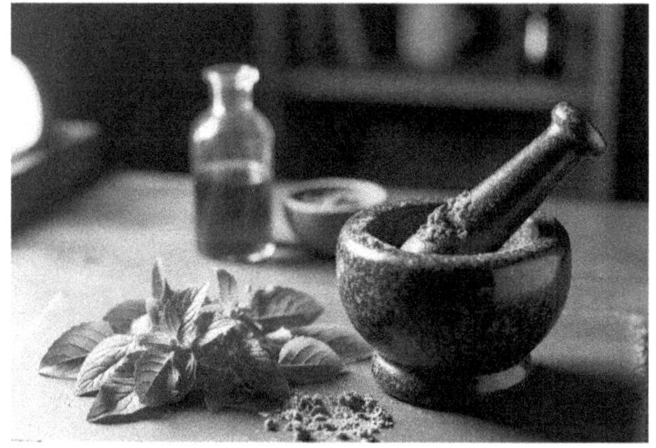

- ***Part Used:*** Leaves

- ***Traditional Uses:*** Diarrhea, stomach cramps

- ***Preparation:*** Pound fresh leaves, boil in 2 cups water for 10 minutes. Strain.

- ***Dosage:*** ½–1 cup daily

- ***Caution:*** Avoid excess

67. Senna (*Cassia angustifolia*)

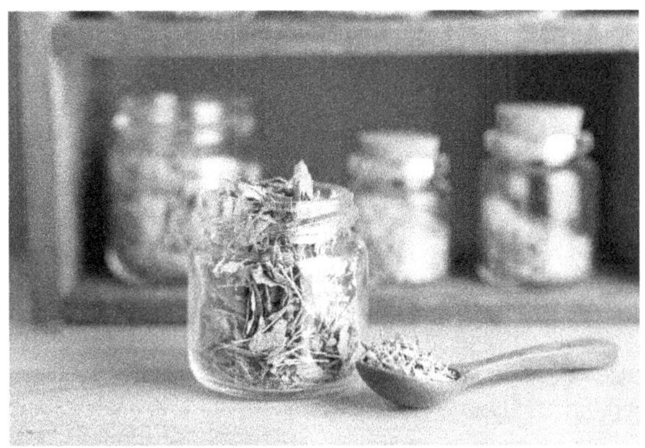

- *Part Used:* Leaves

- *Traditional Uses:* Constipation

- *Preparation:* Steep ½ teaspoon dried leaves in hot water for 5 minutes only. Strain.

- *Dosage:* Once at night

- *Caution:* Do not use more than 3 days

68. Guava Leaf (*Psidium guajava*)

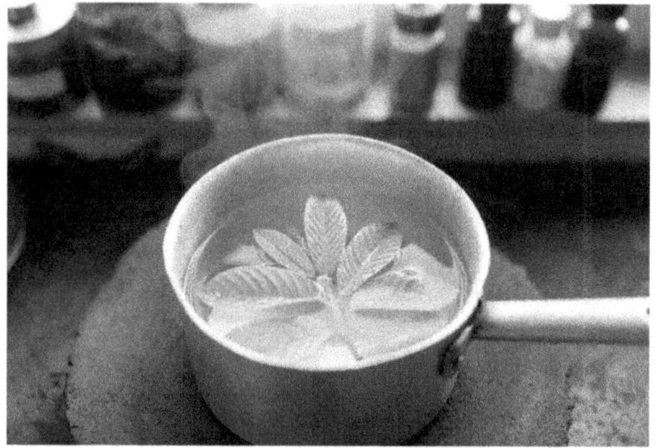

- *Part Used:* Leaves

- *Traditional Uses:* Diarrhea, gut health

- *Preparation:* Boil 5 young leaves in 2 cups water for 10 minutes. Strain.

- *Dosage:* 1 cup twice daily

- *Caution:* Safe short-term

69. Dandelion (*Taraxacum officinale*)

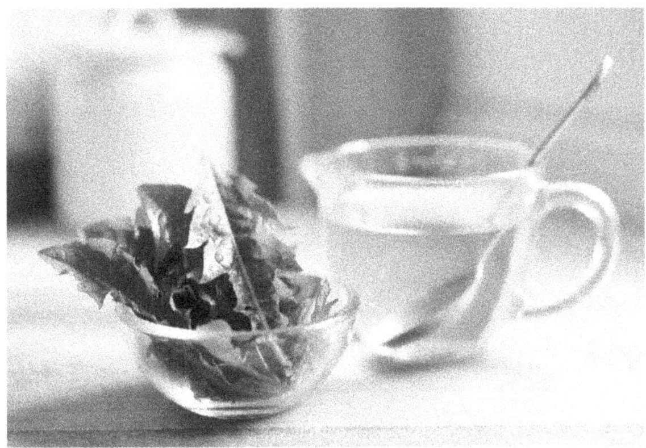

- *Part Used:* Leaves

- *Traditional Uses:* Liver support, detox

- *Preparation:* Wash leaves. Steep 1 tablespoon in hot water for 10 minutes.

- *Dosage:* 1 cup daily

- *Caution:* Avoid bile duct obstruction

70. Pawpaw Leaf (*Carica papaya*)

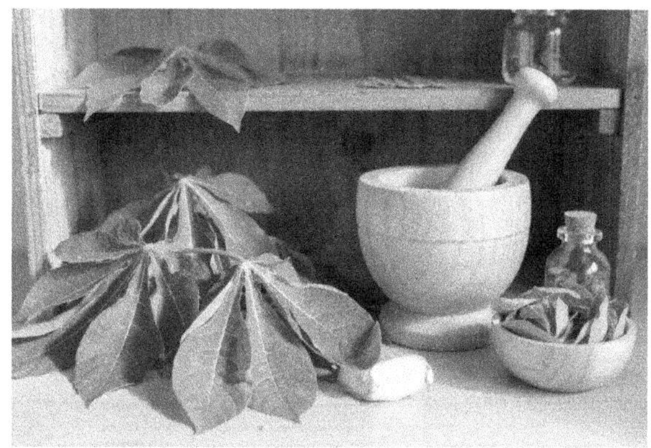

- *Part Used:* Leaves

- *Traditional Uses:* Digestion, malaria support

- *Preparation:* Chop fresh leaves. Boil in 3 cups water for 15 minutes. Strain.

- *Dosage:* ½ cup daily

- *Caution:* Very bitter; avoid excess

71. Lemongrass (*Cymbopogon citratus*)

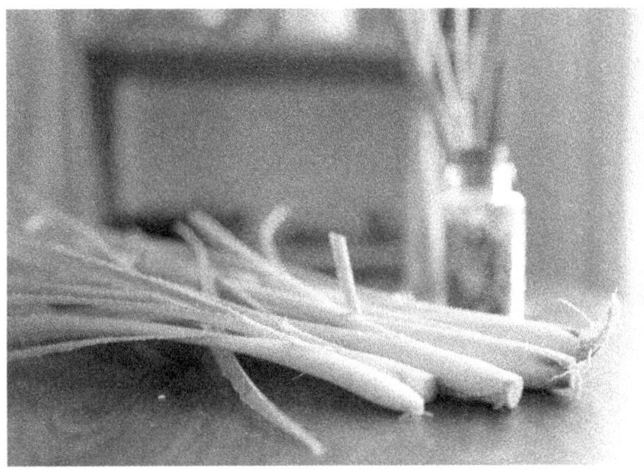

- *Part Used:* Leaves

- *Traditional Uses:* Metabolism, relaxation

- *Preparation:* Cut fresh stalks. Boil 1 stalk in 2 cups water for 10 minutes.

- *Dosage:* 1 cup in the evening

- *Caution:* Avoid low blood pressure

72. Bay Leaf (*Laurus nobilis*)

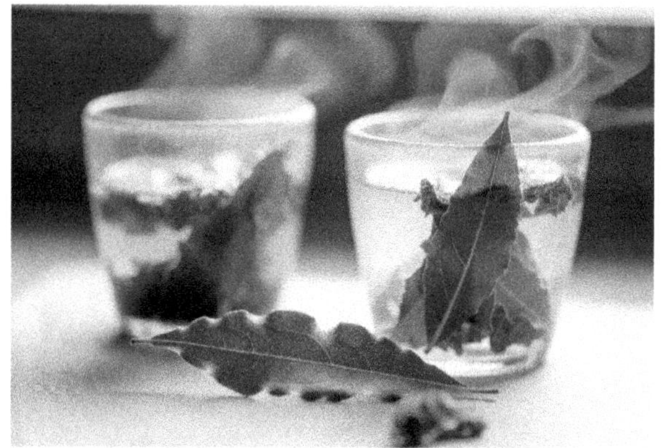

- *Part Used:* Leaves

- *Traditional Uses:* Blood sugar, digestion

- *Preparation:* Boil 2 dried leaves in 2 cups water for 10 minutes. Strain.

- *Dosage:* 1 cup daily

- *Caution:* Do not chew whole leaf

73. Rosemary (*Rosmarinus officinalis*)

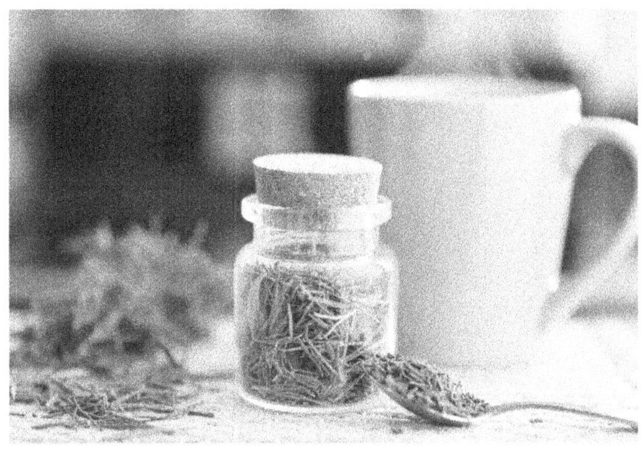

- *Part Used:* Leaves

- *Traditional Uses:* Circulation, memory

- *Preparation:* Steep 1 teaspoon dried leaves in hot water for 10 minutes.

- *Dosage:* 1 cup daily

- *Caution:* Avoid pregnancy

74. Thyme (*Thymus vulgaris*)

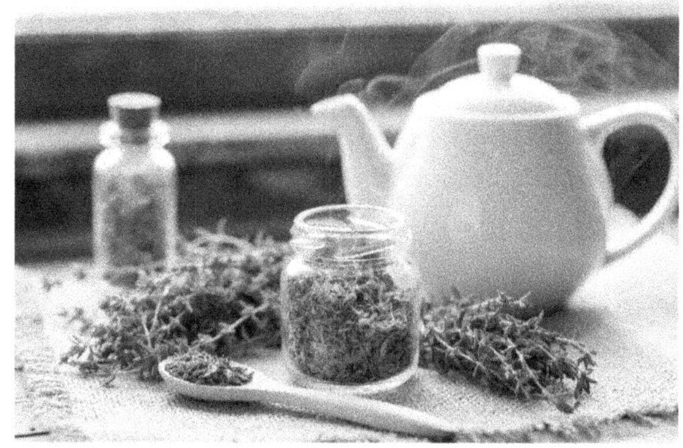

- *Part Used:* Leaves

- *Traditional Uses:* Respiratory and digestion

- *Preparation:* Steep 1 teaspoon dried leaves in boiling water for 7 minutes.

- *Dosage:* 1 cup daily

- *Caution:* Avoid excess

75. Sage (*Salvia officinalis*)

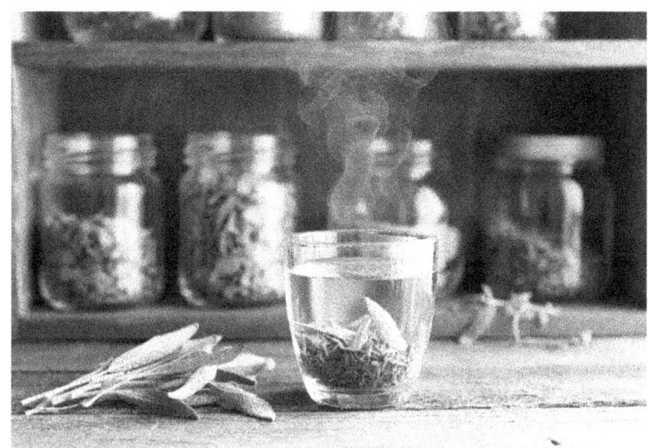

- *Part Used:* Leaves

- *Traditional Uses:* Blood sugar, digestion

- *Preparation:* Steep 1 teaspoon dried leaves in hot water for 10 minutes.

- *Dosage:* 1 cup daily

- *Caution:* Not for long-term use

76. Fluted Pumpkin Leaf (*Telfairia occidentalis*)

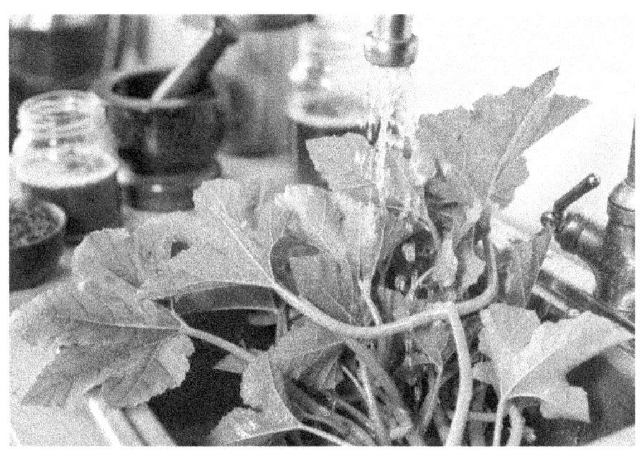

- *Part Used:* Leaves

- *Traditional Uses:* Blood tonic, anemia

- *Preparation:* Wash fresh leaves, blend lightly with water, strain juice.

- *Dosage:* ½ cup fresh juice daily

- *Caution:* Use fresh only

77. Bitter Kola Leaf (*Garcinia kola*)

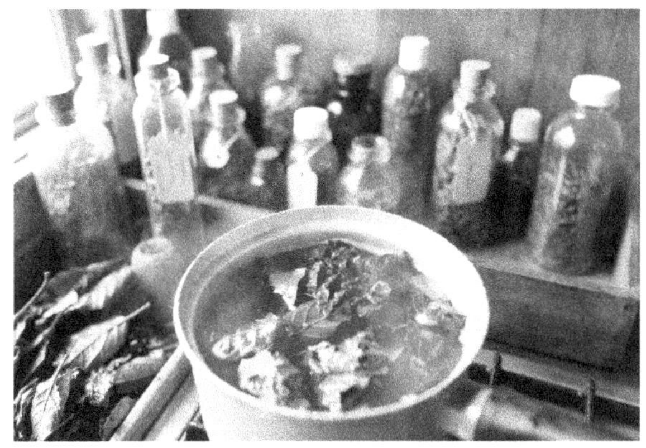

- *Part Used:* Leaves

- *Traditional Uses:* Metabolism, detox

- *Preparation:* Boil chopped leaves in 2 cups water for 15 minutes. Strain.

- *Dosage:* ½ cup daily

- *Caution:* Avoid excess

78. Plantain Leaf (*Plantago major*)

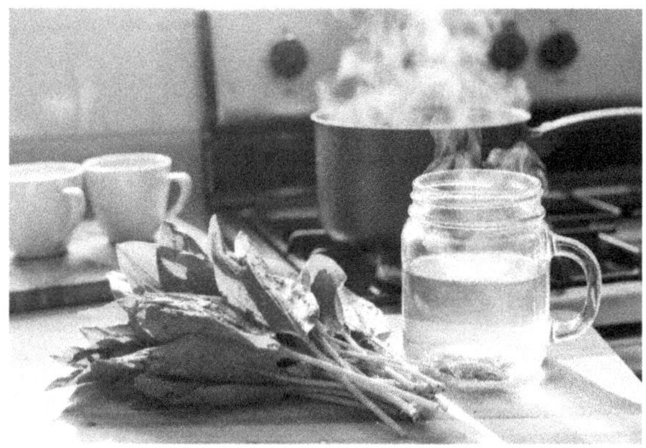

- *Part Used:* Leaves

- *Traditional Uses:* Gut inflammation

- *Preparation:* Wash leaves. Boil in 2 cups water for 10 minutes. Strain.

- *Dosage:* 1 cup daily

- *Caution:* Safe short-term

79. Nettle (*Urtica dioica*)

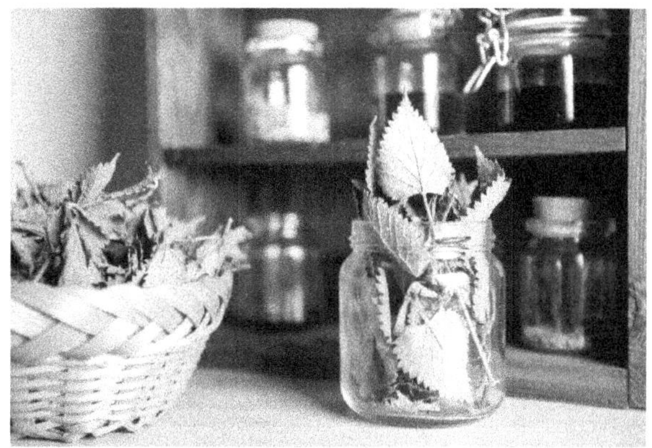

- *Part Used:* Leaves

- *Traditional Uses:* Blood building, detox

- *Preparation:* Dry leaves first. Steep 1 tablespoon in hot water for 10 minutes.

- *Dosage:* 1 cup daily

- *Caution:* Avoid kidney disease

80. Hibiscus Leaf (*Hibiscus sabdariffa*)

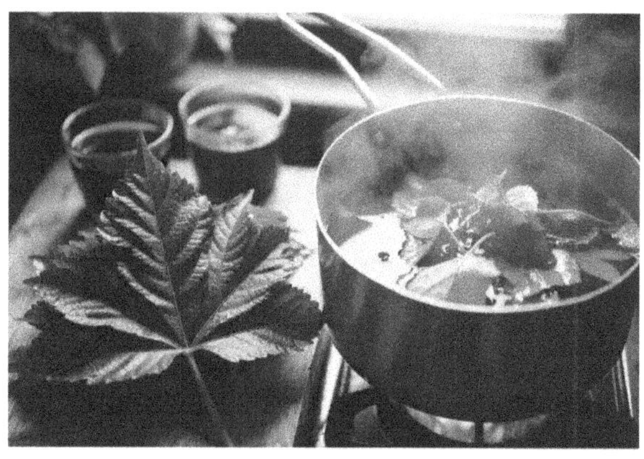

- *Part Used:* Leaves

- *Traditional Uses:* Metabolism, blood pressure

- *Preparation:* Boil fresh leaves in 2 cups water for 10 minutes. Strain.

- *Dosage:* 1 cup daily

- *Caution:* Monitor blood pressure

Next section: Remedies 81–100

Liver, Kidney & Detox-support Leaves (81–100)

81. Bitter Leaf (*Vernonia amygdalina*)

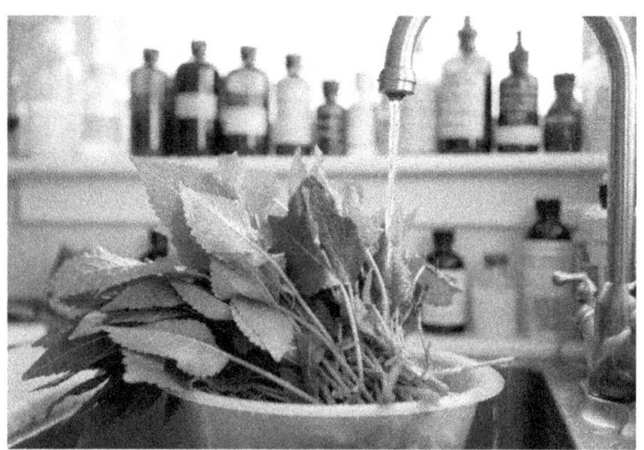

- *Part Used:* Leaves

- *Traditional Uses:* Liver detox, blood sugar support

- *Preparation:*

1. Wash leaves thoroughly and squeeze repeatedly to reduce bitterness.

2. Boil lightly in clean water for 5–7 minutes.

3. Strain and drink warm.

- *Dosage:* ½ cup daily

- *Caution:* Excess bitterness may cause nausea

82. Neem Leaf (*Azadirachta indica*)

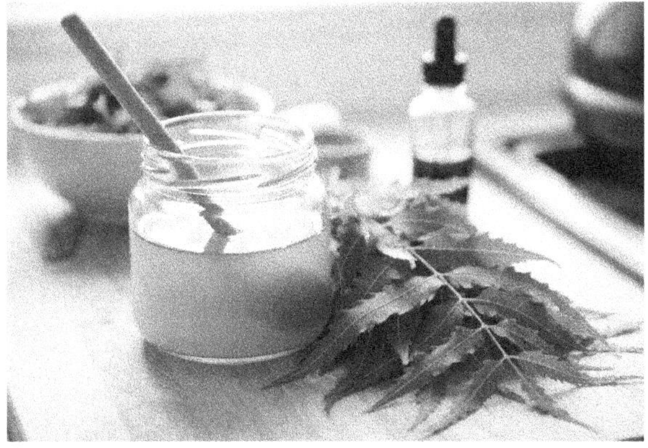

- *Part Used:* Leaves

- *Traditional Uses:* Liver cleansing, infections

- *Preparation:* Decoction (simmer leaves for 10 minutes)

- *Dosage:* Small cup daily

- *Caution:* Avoid pregnancy

83. Dandelion Leaf (*Taraxacum officinale*)

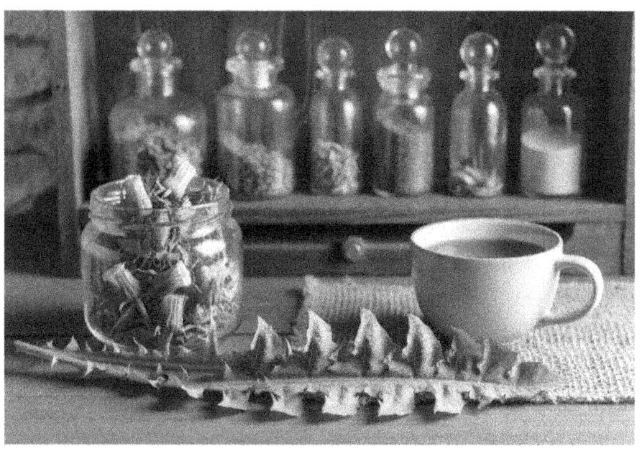

- *Part Used:* Leaves

- *Traditional Uses:* Kidney cleansing, diuretic

- *Preparation:* Tea (steep dried leaves in hot water)

- *Dosage:* 1 cup daily

- *Caution:* Avoid bile obstruction

84. Senna Leaf (*Senna alexandrina*)

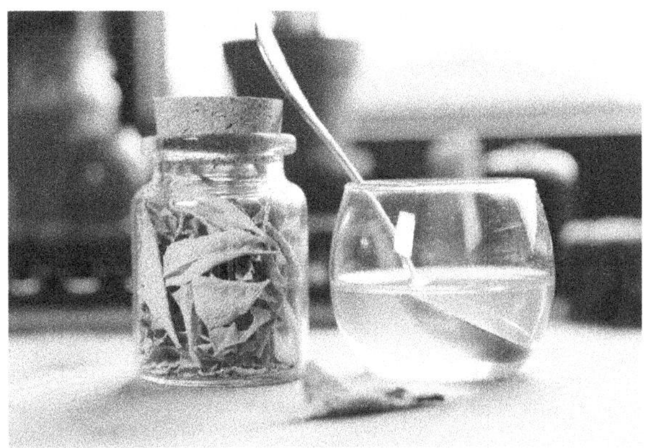

- *Part Used:* Leaves

- *Traditional Uses:* Constipation, bowel cleansing

- *Preparation:* Light tea infusion (steep briefly)

- *Dosage:* Short-term use only

- *Caution:* Not for long-term use

85. Chanca Piedra (*Phyllanthus niruri*)

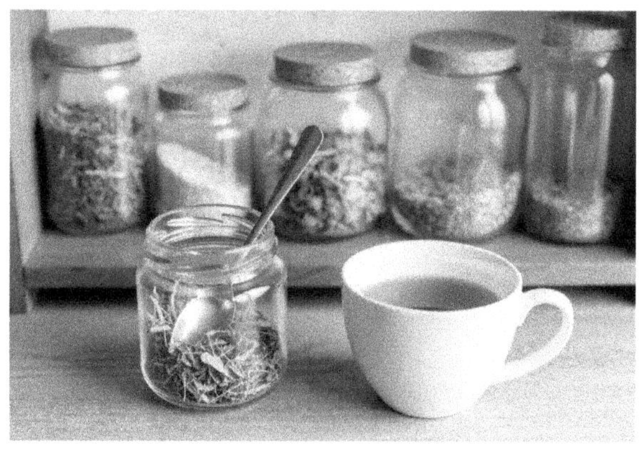

- *Part Used:* Whole plant
- *Traditional Uses:* Kidney stones, liver support
- *Preparation:* Decoction
- *Dosage:* 1 cup daily
- *Caution:* Avoid pregnancy

86. Pawpaw Leaf (*Carica papaya*)

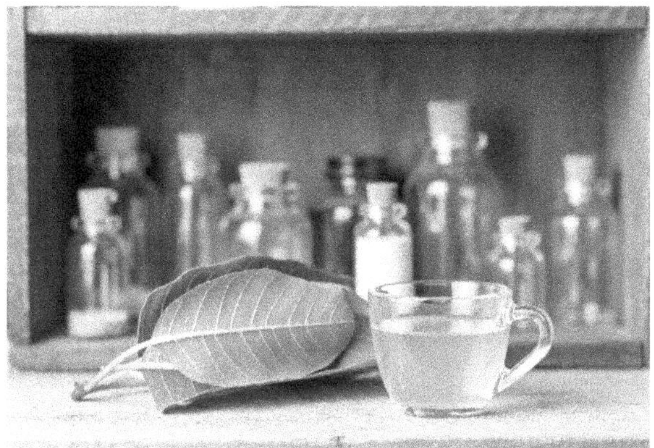

- *Part Used:* Leaves

- *Traditional Uses:* Liver cleansing, platelet support

- *Preparation:* Fresh juice or mild decoction

- *Dosage:* 1 tablespoon juice daily

- *Caution:* Very bitter

87. Guava Leaf (*Psidium guajava*)

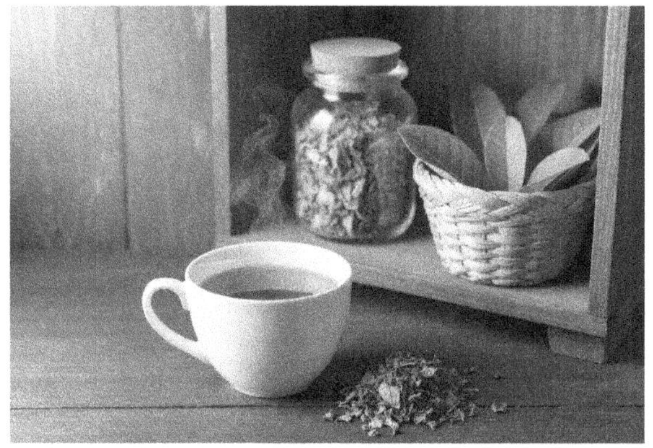

- ***Part Used:*** Leaves

- ***Traditional Uses:*** Diarrhea, detox

- ***Preparation:*** Tea

- ***Dosage:*** 1 cup daily

- ***Caution:*** None known

88. Plantain Leaf (*Plantago major*)

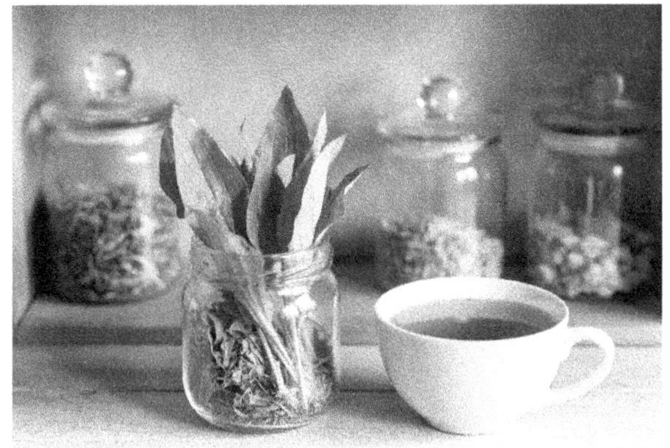

- *Part Used:* Leaves

- *Traditional Uses:* Kidney support, urinary health

- *Preparation:* Tea

- *Dosage:* 1 cup daily

- *Caution:* Correct identification required

89. Boldo Leaf (*Peumus boldus*)

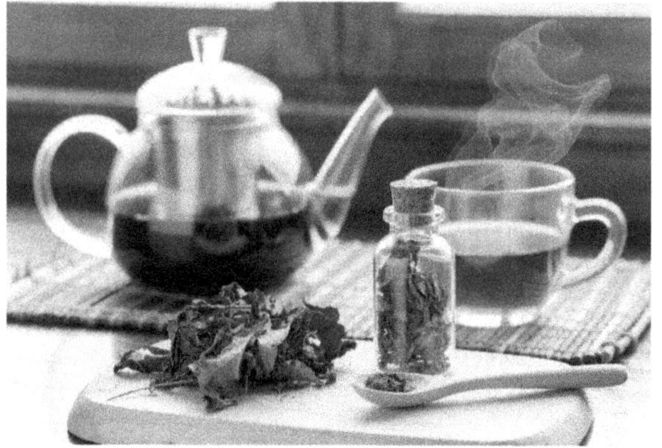

- *Part Used:* Leaves

- *Traditional Uses:* Liver stimulation

- *Preparation:* Tea

- *Dosage:* Small cup daily

- *Caution:* Avoid pregnancy

90. Artichoke Leaf (*Cynara scolymus*)

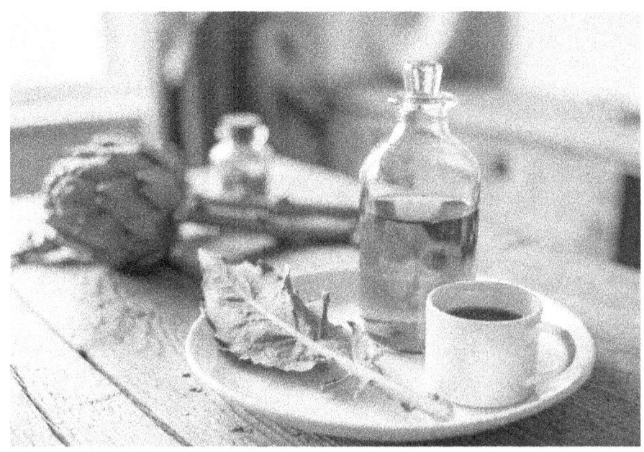

- *Part Used:* Leaves

- *Traditional Uses:* Liver detox, cholesterol support

- *Preparation:* Tea or extract

- *Dosage:* 1 cup daily

- *Caution:* Gallstones

91. Milk Thistle Leaf (*Silybum marianum*)

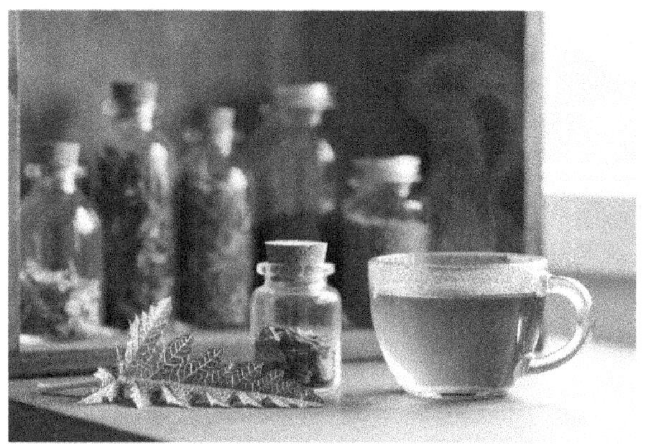

- *Part Used:* Leaves

- *Traditional Uses:* Liver protection

- *Preparation:* Tea

- *Dosage:* 1 cup daily

- *Caution:* Allergy risk

92. Cassava Leaf (*Manihot esculenta*)

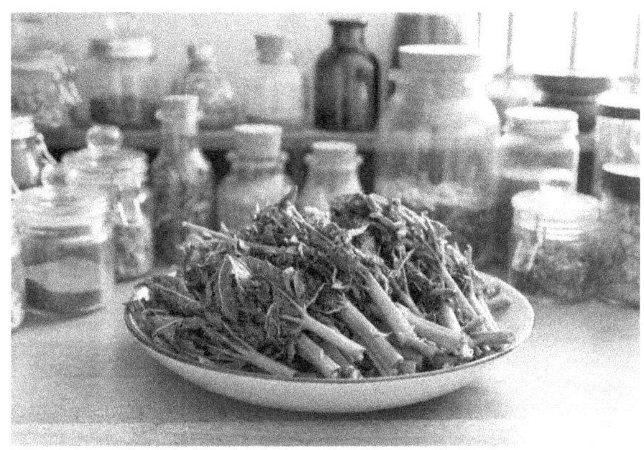

- *Part Used:* Leaves

- *Traditional Uses:* Detox, nutrition

- *Preparation:* Thoroughly cooked as vegetable

- *Dosage:* As food

- *Caution:* Never consume raw

93. Mustard Green (*Brassica juncea*)

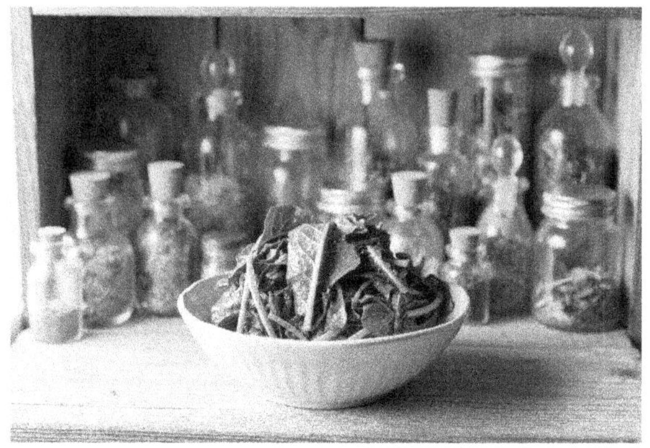

- *Part Used:* Leaves

- *Traditional Uses:* Detox, digestion

- *Preparation:* Lightly steamed

- *Dosage:* As food

- *Caution:* Avoid excess

94. Kale (*Brassica oleracea*)

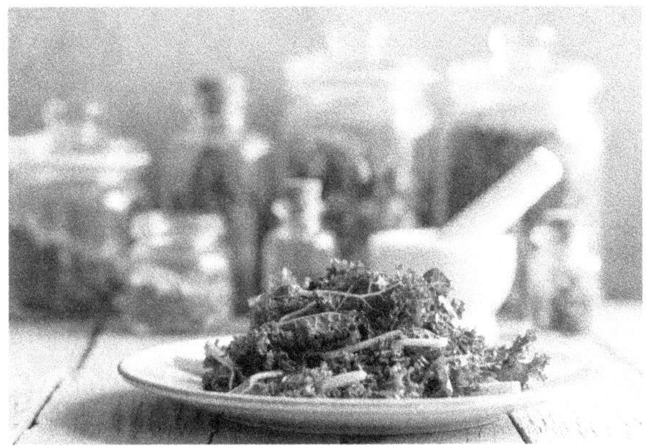

- *Part Used:* Leaves

- *Traditional Uses:* Liver enzyme support

- *Preparation:* Lightly cooked

- *Dosage:* As food

- *Caution:* Avoid excess raw intake

95. Watercress (*Nasturtium officinale*)

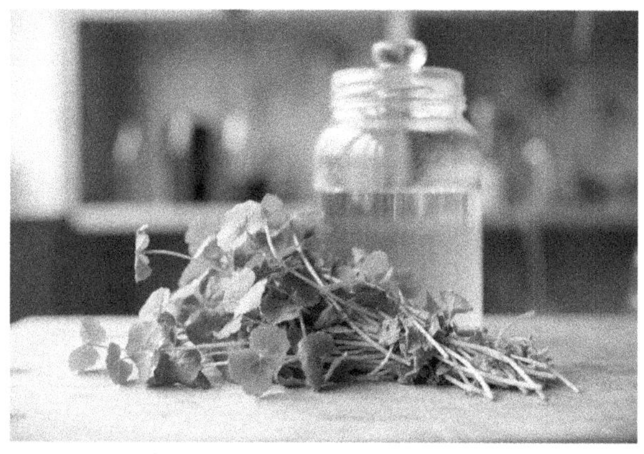

- *Part Used:* Leaves

- *Traditional Uses:* Kidney cleansing

- *Preparation:* Fresh or tea

- *Dosage:* As food

- *Caution:* Wash thoroughly

96. Coriander Leaf (*Coriandrum sativum*)

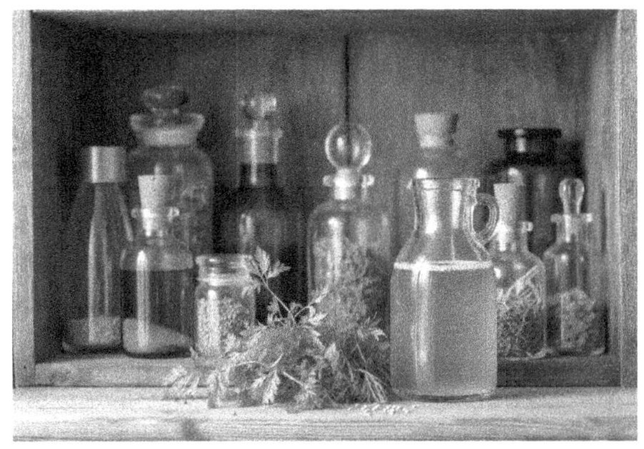

- *Part Used:* Leaves
- *Traditional Uses:* Heavy metal detox support
- *Preparation:* Juice or tea
- *Dosage:* Small cup daily
- *Caution:* Mild diuretic

97. Celosia Leaf (*Celosia argentea*)

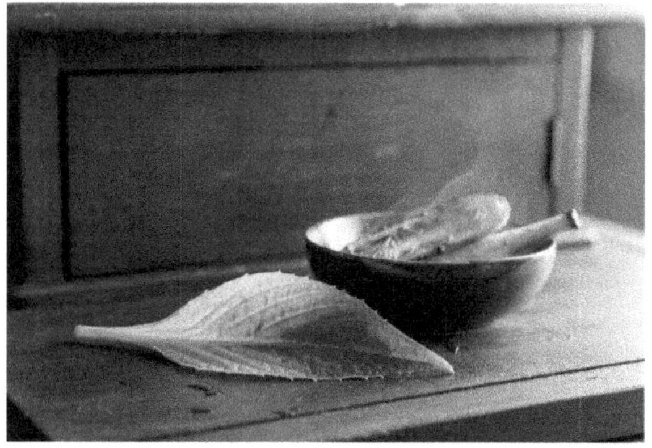

- *Part Used:* Leaves

- *Traditional Uses:* Liver health, digestion

- *Preparation:* Cooked vegetable

- *Dosage:* As food

- *Caution:* None known

98. Holy Basil (*Ocimum sanctum*)

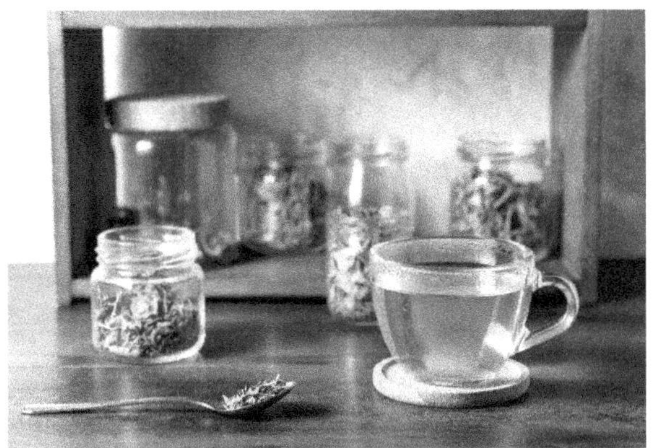

- *Part Used:* Leaves

- *Traditional Uses:* Liver protection, stress support

- *Preparation:* Tea

- *Dosage:* 1 cup daily

- *Caution:* Avoid excess

99. Bay Leaf (*Laurus nobilis*)

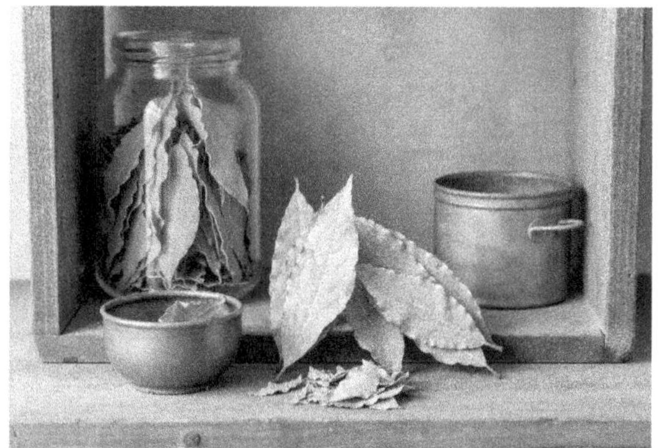

- *Part Used:* Leaves

- *Traditional Uses:* Detox, digestion

- *Preparation:* Tea or cooking spice

- *Dosage:* 1 cup tea daily

- *Caution:* Remove leaf before consumption

100. Soursop Leaf (*Annona muricata*)

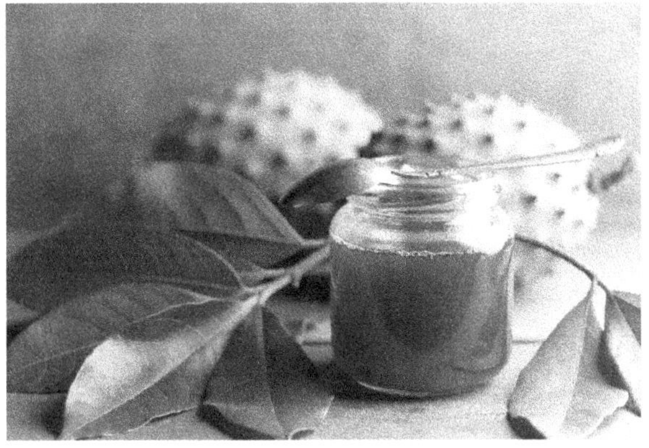

- *Part Used:* Leaves

- *Traditional Uses:* Liver cleansing, immune support

- *Preparation:* Decoction (simmer for 10–15 minutes)

- *Dosage:* ½–1 cup daily

- *Caution:* Avoid prolonged continuous use

Respiratory, Cold & Fever-support Leaves (101–120)

101. Eucalyptus (*Eucalyptus globulus*)

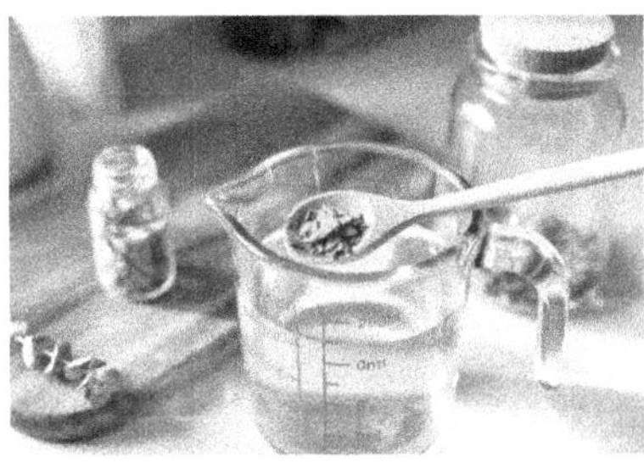

- *Part Used:* Leaves

- *Traditional Uses:* Respiratory congestion, colds, cough

- *Preparation:*

1. Boil 1 tablespoon of dried eucalyptus leaves in 2 cups of water.

2. Simmer for 10 minutes.

3. Strain the infusion.

4. Drink warm or inhale the steam for congestion relief.

- *Dosage:* 1 cup up to 3 times daily

- *Caution:* Not for children under 12; avoid ingestion of essential oil

102. Peppermint (*Mentha piperita*)

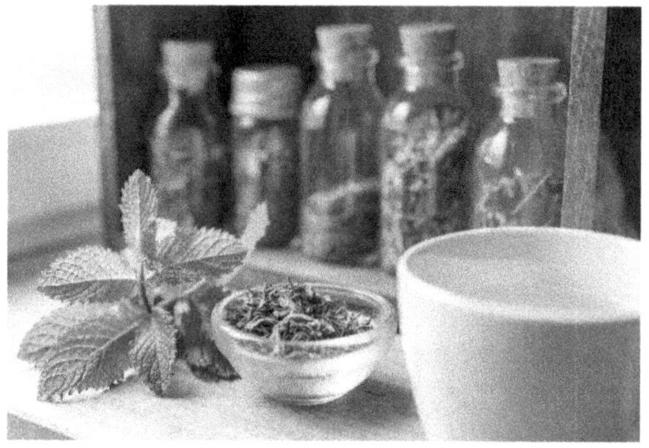

- ***Part Used:*** Leaves

- ***Traditional Uses:*** Nasal congestion, headache, digestive issues

- ***Preparation:***

1. Steep 1 tablespoon of fresh or dried peppermint leaves in 1 cup boiling water.

2. Cover and steep for 7–10 minutes.

3. Strain and drink warm.

- ***Dosage:*** 1–2 cups daily

- ***Caution:*** Avoid if prone to acid reflux

103. Lemon Balm (*Melissa officinalis*)

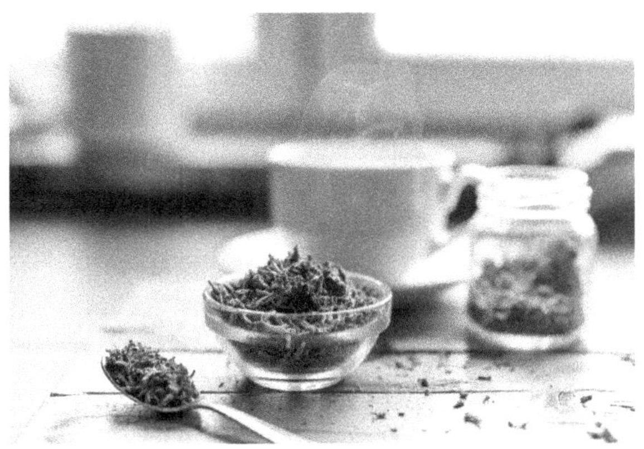

- *Part Used:* Leaves

- *Traditional Uses:* Cold sores, fever, anxiety

- *Preparation:*

1. Infuse 1 tablespoon of dried lemon balm leaves in 1 cup hot water.

2. Steep for 10 minutes.

3. Strain and drink.

- *Dosage:* Up to 3 cups daily

- *Caution:* May cause drowsiness; avoid excessive use

104. Thyme (*Thymus vulgaris*)

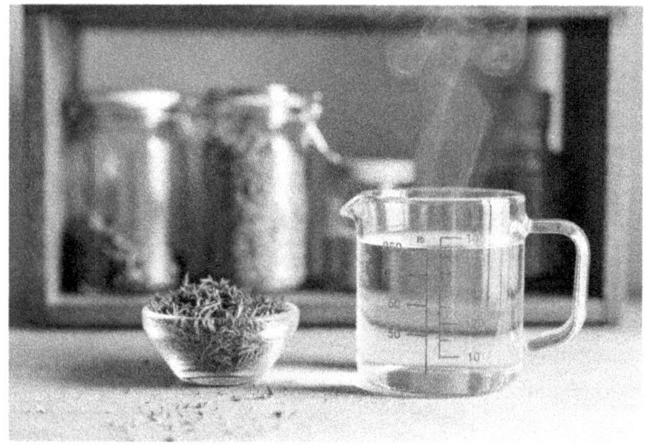

- *Part Used:* Leaves

- *Traditional Uses:* Cough, bronchitis, respiratory infections

- *Preparation:*

1. Add 1 teaspoon of dried thyme leaves to 1 cup boiling water.

2. Cover and steep for 10 minutes.

3. Strain and drink warm.

- *Dosage:* 1–2 cups daily

- *Caution:* Avoid high doses during pregnancy

105. Mullein (*Verbascum thapsus*)

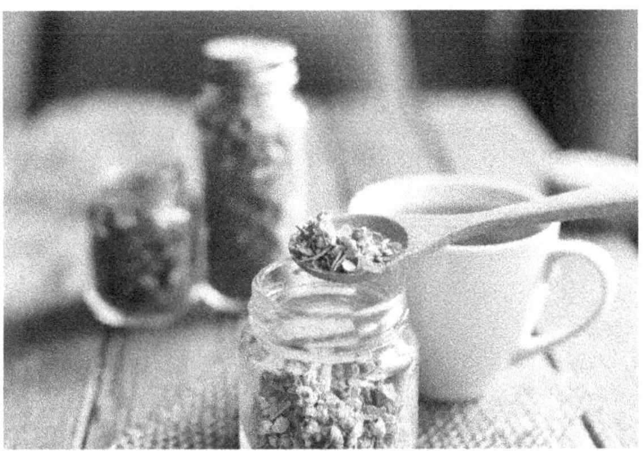

- ***Part Used:*** Leaves and flowers

- ***Traditional Uses:*** Cough, bronchitis, lung health

- ***Preparation:***

1. Steep 1 tablespoon of dried leaves or flowers in 1 cup hot water.

2. Cover and let steep for 10 minutes.

3. Strain and drink warm.

- ***Dosage:*** 1–3 cups daily

- ***Caution:*** Avoid if allergic to plants in the fig family

106. Elderberry (*Sambucus nigra*)

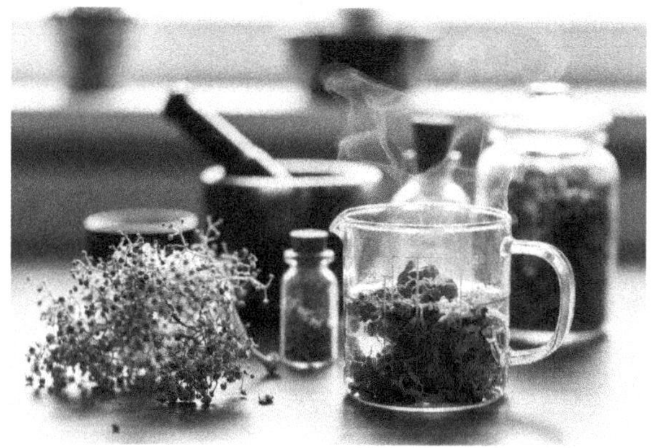

- *Part Used:* Leaves and flowers (flowers commonly used)

- *Traditional Uses:* Cold, flu, immune support

- *Preparation:*

1. Steep 1 tablespoon of dried elderflowers in 1 cup boiling water.

2. Cover and steep for 10 minutes.

3. Strain and drink warm.

- *Dosage:* 1–2 cups daily during illness

- *Caution:* Raw berries and other parts are toxic if not cooked

107. Sage (*Salvia officinalis*)

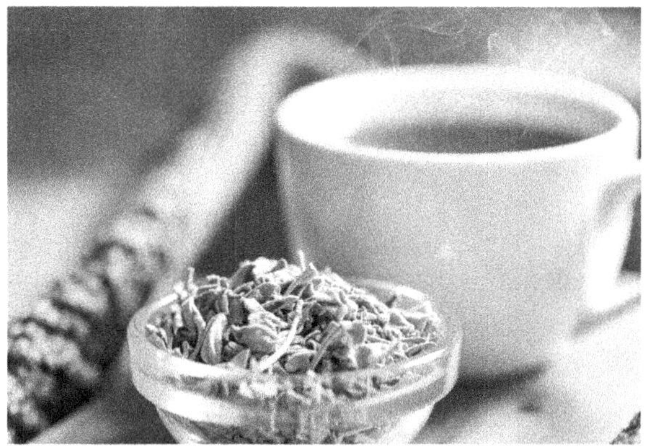

- *Part Used:* Leaves

- *Traditional Uses:* Sore throat, cough, inflammation

- *Preparation:*

1. Infuse 1 tablespoon of dried sage leaves in 1 cup hot water.

2. Steep for 10 minutes.

3. Strain and use as a tea or gargle.

- *Dosage:* 1 cup up to 3 times daily

- *Caution:* Avoid prolonged use; may be toxic in high doses

108. Echinacea (*Echinacea purpurea*)

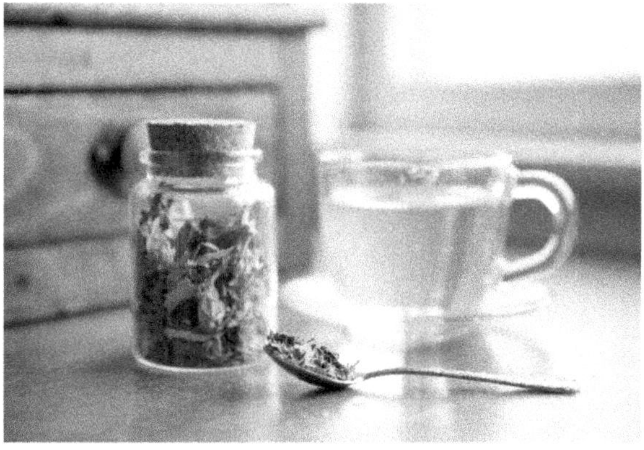

- *Part Used:* Leaves and roots

- *Traditional Uses:* Immune support, cold, flu

- *Preparation:*

1. Simmer 1 teaspoon of dried root or leaves in 1 cup water for 10 minutes.

2. Strain and drink warm.

- *Dosage:* 1 cup up to 3 times daily

- *Caution:* Allergic reactions possible; avoid if autoimmune conditions

109. Coltsfoot (*Tussilago farfara*)

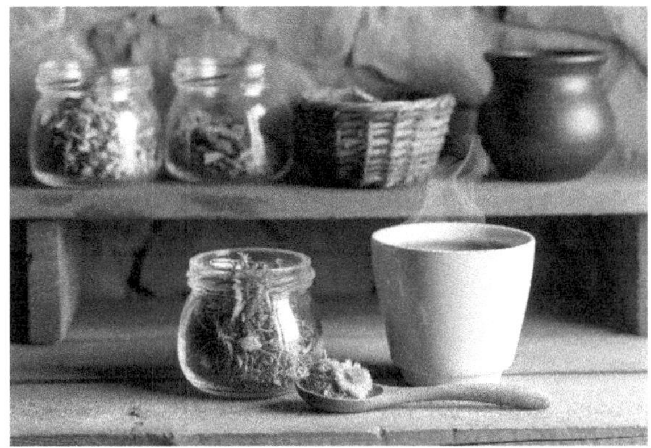

- *Part Used:* Leaves and flowers

- *Traditional Uses:* Cough, bronchitis, respiratory relief

- *Preparation:*

1. Steep 1 tablespoon dried leaves or flowers in 1 cup boiling water.

2. Cover and steep for 10 minutes.

3. Strain and drink warm.

- *Dosage:* 1–2 cups daily

- *Caution:* Avoid prolonged use due to liver toxicity risk

110. Plantain Leaf (*Plantago major*)

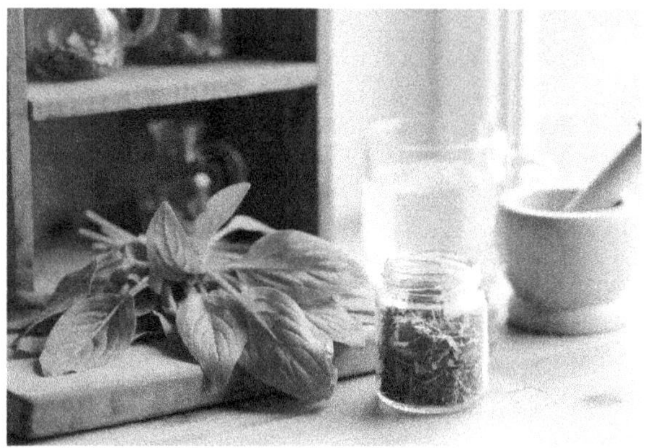

- *Part Used:* Leaves

- *Traditional Uses:* Cough, throat irritation, wound healing

- *Preparation:*

1. Crush fresh leaves or steep dried leaves in hot water.

2. For tea: steep 1 tablespoon dried leaves in 1 cup water for 10 minutes.

3. Strain and drink warm.

- *Dosage:* 1 cup up to 3 times daily

- *Caution:* Ensure proper identification

111. Licorice (*Glycyrrhiza glabra*)

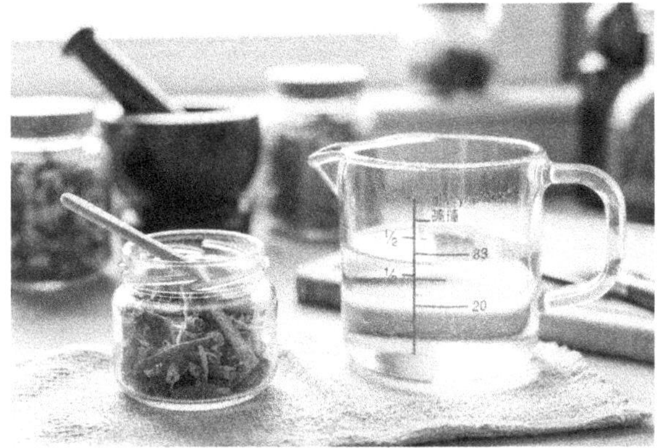

- *Part Used:* Root

- *Traditional Uses:* Soothing sore throat, cough, adrenal support

- *Preparation:*

1. Simmer 1 teaspoon dried root in 1 1/2 cups water for 10 minutes.

2. Strain and drink warm.

- *Dosage:* 1 cup up to twice daily

- *Caution:* Avoid prolonged use in hypertension

112. Marshmallow Root (*Althaea officinalis*)

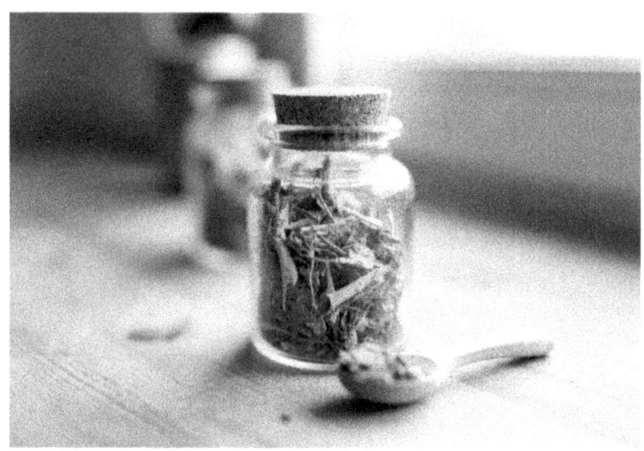

- ***Part Used:*** Root

- ***Traditional Uses:*** Soothing mucous membranes, cough, throat irritation

- ***Preparation:***

1. Soak 1 tablespoon dried root in cold water for 8 hours or overnight.

2. Heat gently without boiling.

3. Strain and drink warm.

- ***Dosage:*** 1 cup up to 3 times daily

- ***Caution:*** May affect absorption of other medicines

113. Anise (*Pimpinella anisum*)

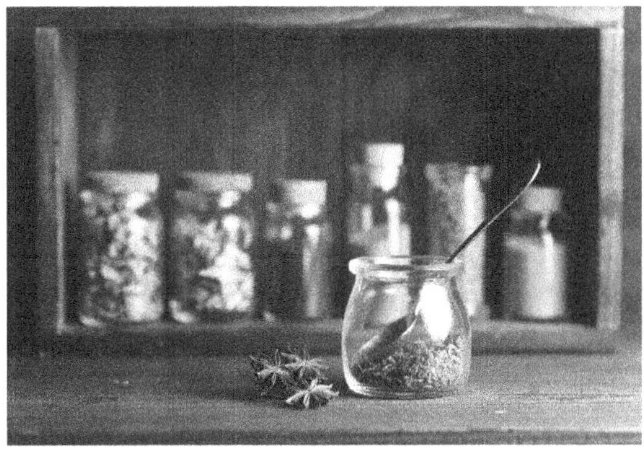

- *Part Used:* Seeds

- *Traditional Uses:* Cough, bronchitis, digestive aid

- *Preparation:*

1. Crush 1 teaspoon seeds lightly.

2. Steep in 1 cup boiling water for 10 minutes.

3. Strain and drink warm.

- *Dosage:* 1 cup up to twice daily

- *Caution:* Avoid in case of allergy to plants in the carrot family

114. Horehound (*Marrubium vulgare*)

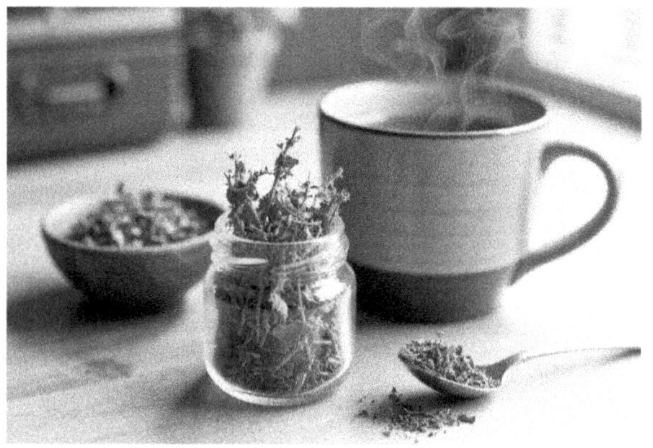

- *Part Used:* Leaves

- *Traditional Uses:* Cough, bronchitis, expectorant

- *Preparation:*

1. Steep 1 tablespoon dried leaves in 1 cup boiling water.

2. Cover and steep for 10 minutes.

3. Strain and drink warm.

- *Dosage:* 1–2 cups daily

- *Caution:* Avoid during pregnancy

115. Eucalyptus (*Eucalyptus radiata*)

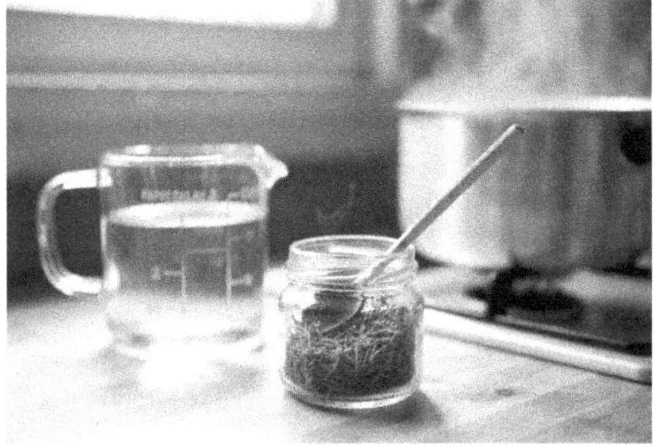

- ***Part Used:*** Leaves

- ***Traditional Uses:*** Respiratory congestion, cold relief

- ***Preparation:***

1. Boil 1 teaspoon dried leaves in 2 cups water.

2. Simmer for 10 minutes.

3. Strain and drink or inhale steam.

- ***Dosage:*** 1 cup up to 3 times daily

- ***Caution:*** Not for children orally

116. Coltsfoot (*Tussilago farfara*)

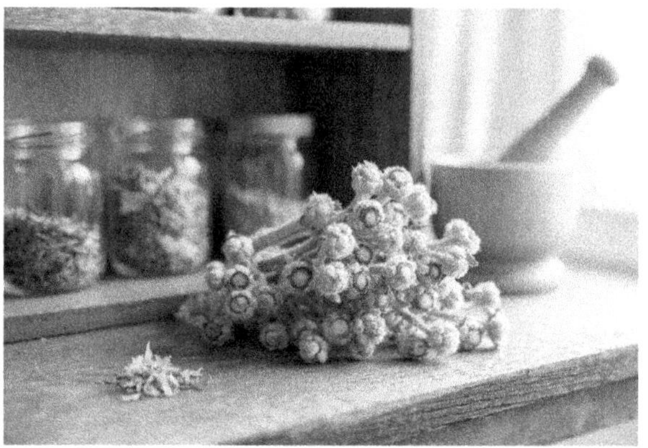

- *Part Used:* Leaves and flowers

- *Traditional Uses:* Cough, bronchitis

- *Preparation:*

1. Steep 1 tablespoon dried leaves or flowers in 1 cup boiling water.

2. Cover and steep for 10 minutes.

3. Strain and drink warm.

- *Dosage:* 1–2 cups daily

- *Caution:* Use short term only

117. Ginger (*Zingiber officinale*)

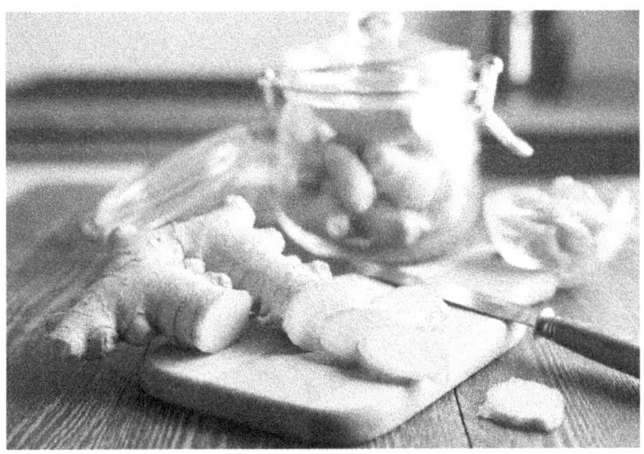

- ***Part Used:*** Rhizome

- ***Traditional Uses:*** Cold, cough, warming, anti-inflammatory

- ***Preparation:***

1. Slice 5–6 fresh ginger pieces.

2. Add 1 1/2 cups boiling water.

3. Steep for 10 minutes.

4. Strain and drink warm.

- ***Dosage:*** 1–2 cups daily

- ***Caution:*** Avoid excess with ulcers

118. Lemon Grass (*Cymbopogon citratus*)

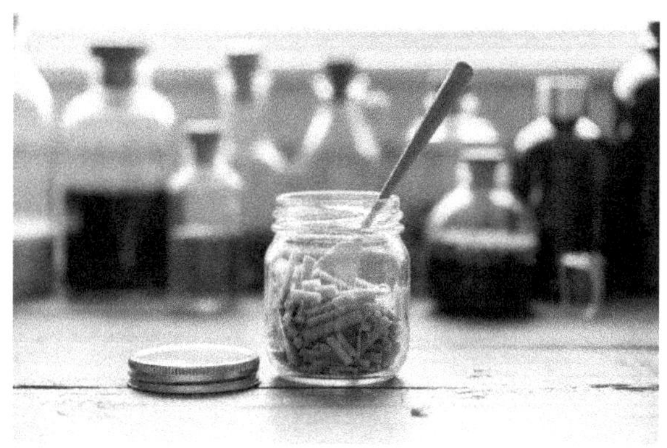

- ***Part Used:*** Leaves

- ***Traditional Uses:*** Fever, cold, digestion

- ***Preparation:***

1. Chop 1 tablespoon fresh lemongrass.

2. Boil in 2 cups water for 10 minutes.

3. Strain and drink warm.

- ***Dosage:*** 1–2 cups daily

- ***Caution:*** May lower blood pressure

119. Raspberry Leaf (*Rubus idaeus*)

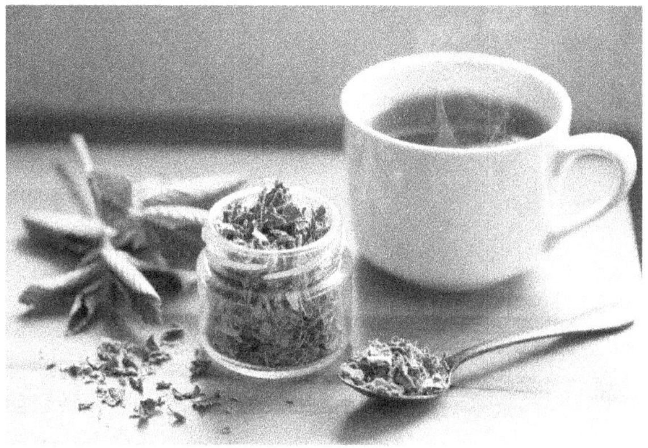

- *Part Used:* Leaves

- *Traditional Uses:* Cough, respiratory support

- *Preparation:*

1. Steep 1 tablespoon dried leaves in 1 cup boiling water.

2. Cover and steep for 10 minutes.

3. Strain and drink warm.

- *Dosage:* 1–2 cups daily

- *Caution:* Avoid during pregnancy

120. Horehound (*Marrubium vulgare*)

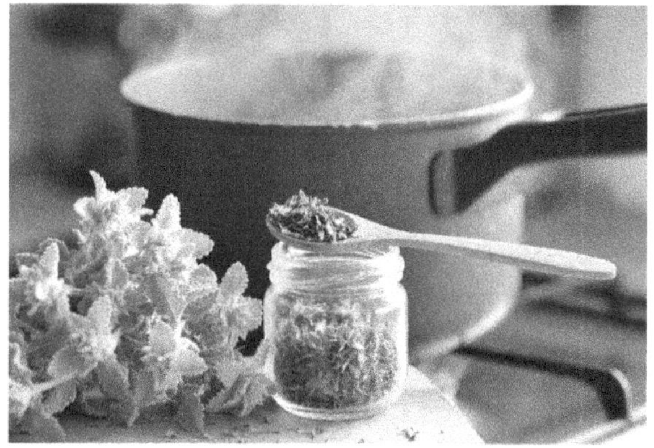

- ***Part Used:*** Leaves

- ***Traditional Uses:*** Cough, bronchitis, expectorant

- ***Preparation:***

1. Steep 1 tablespoon dried leaves in 1 cup boiling water.

2. Cover and steep for 10 minutes.

3. Strain and drink warm.

- ***Dosage:*** 1–2 cups daily

- ***Caution:*** Avoid during pregnancy

Nervous System, Sleep & Stress-support Leaves (121–140)

121. Valerian (*Valeriana officinalis*)

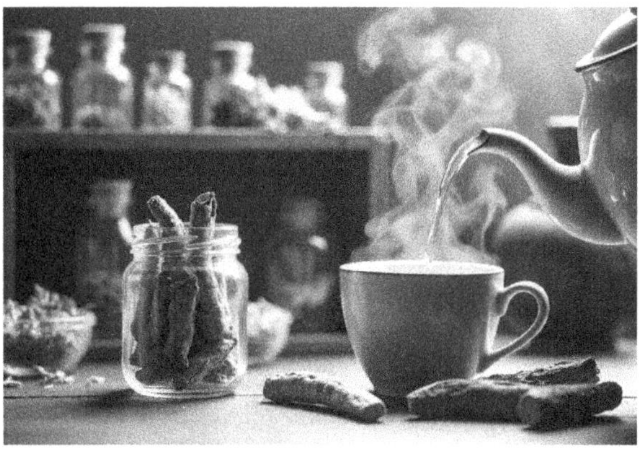

- *Part Used:* Root

- *Traditional Uses:* Insomnia, anxiety, nervous tension

- *Preparation:*

1. Add 1 teaspoon dried valerian root to 1 cup boiling water.

2. Cover and steep for 10–15 minutes.

3. Strain and drink warm.

- *Dosage:* 1 cup 30 minutes before bedtime

- *Caution:* May cause drowsiness; avoid with sedatives

122. Passionflower (*Passiflora incarnata*)

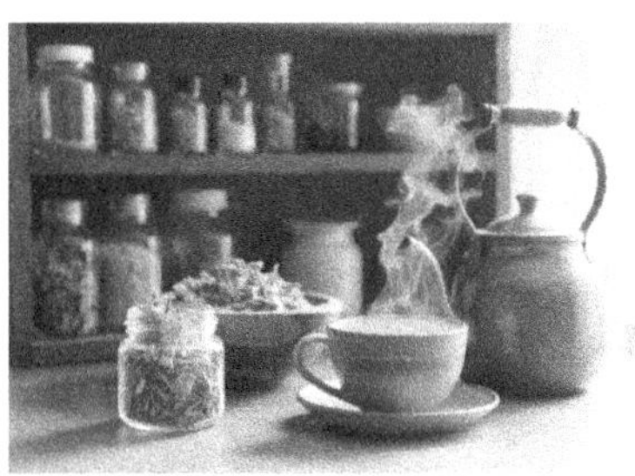

- *Part Used:* Aerial parts (leaves, stems, flowers)

- *Traditional Uses:* Anxiety, insomnia, nervous restlessness

- *Preparation:*

1. Steep 1 tablespoon dried passionflower in 1 cup boiling water.

2. Cover and steep for 10 minutes.

3. Strain and drink.

- *Dosage:* 1–2 cups daily

- *Caution:* Avoid in pregnancy; may cause dizziness

123. Lemon Balm (*Melissa officinalis*)

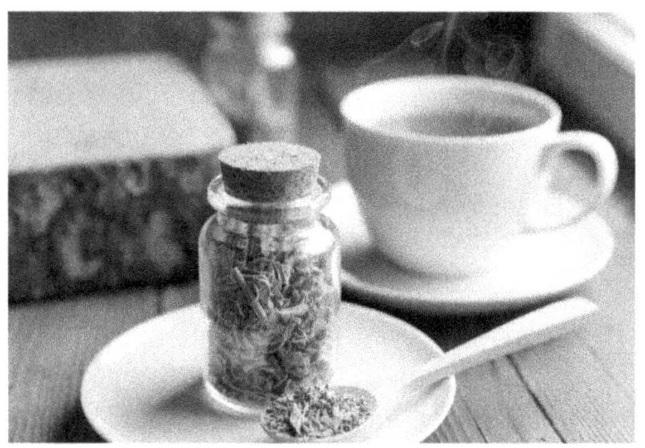

- *Part Used:* Leaves

- *Traditional Uses:* Stress, anxiety, sleep aid

- *Preparation:*

1. Infuse 1 tablespoon dried lemon balm leaves in 1 cup hot water.

2. Steep for 10 minutes.

3. Strain and drink warm.

- *Dosage:* Up to 3 cups daily

- *Caution:* May cause drowsiness

124. Chamomile (*Matricaria chamomilla*)

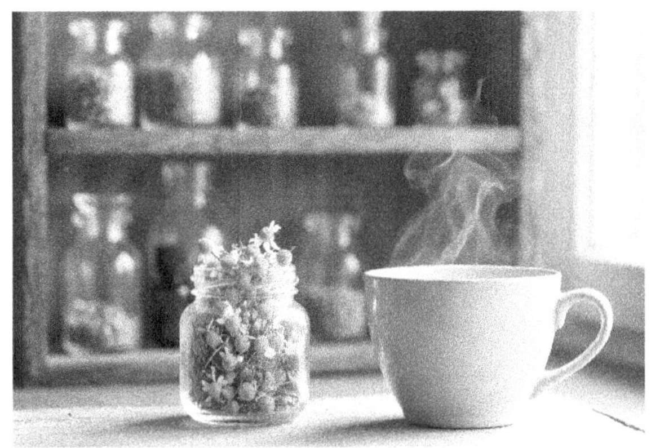

- *Part Used:* Flowers

- *Traditional Uses:* Sleep, anxiety, digestion

- *Preparation:*

1. Steep 1 tablespoon dried chamomile flowers in 1 cup boiling water.

2. Cover and steep for 10 minutes.

3. Strain and drink warm.

- *Dosage:* 1 cup before bedtime

- *Caution:* Allergy risk for ragweed-sensitive individuals

125. Skullcap (*Scutellaria lateriflora*)

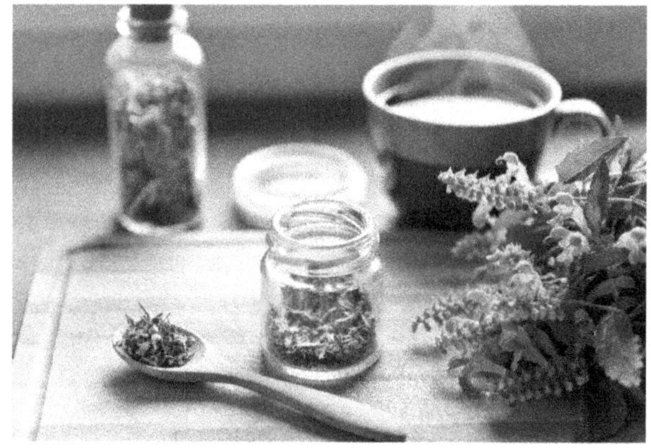

- *Part Used:* Aerial parts

- *Traditional Uses:* Nervous tension, insomnia

- *Preparation:*

1. Steep 1 teaspoon dried skullcap in 1 cup boiling water.

2. Cover and steep for 10 minutes.

3. Strain and drink.

- *Dosage:* 1–2 cups daily

- *Caution:* Avoid long-term use

126. Hops (*Humulus lupulus*)

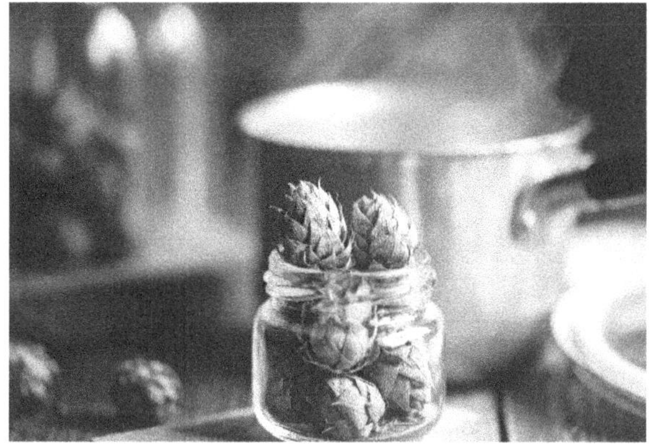

- *Part Used:* Flower cones

- *Traditional Uses:* Insomnia, anxiety

- *Preparation:*

1. Steep 1 tablespoon dried hop cones in 1 cup boiling water.

2. Cover and steep for 10 minutes.

3. Strain and drink warm.

- *Dosage:* 1 cup before bedtime

- *Caution:* May cause allergic reactions

127. Lavender (*Lavandula angustifolia*)

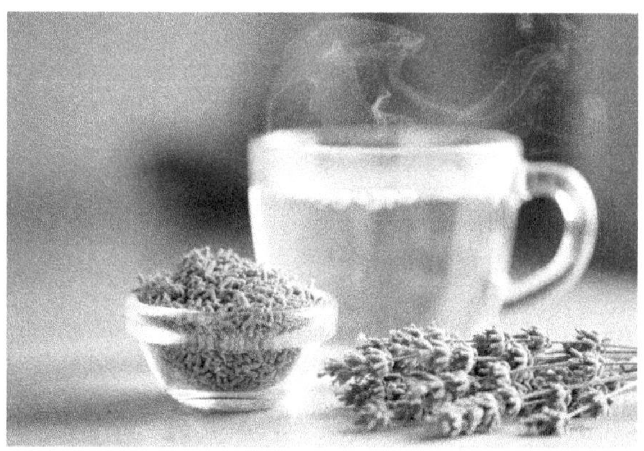

- *Part Used:* Flowers

- *Traditional Uses:* Anxiety, insomnia, mood support

- *Preparation:*

1. Steep 1 tablespoon dried lavender flowers in 1 cup boiling water.

2. Cover and steep for 10 minutes.

3. Strain and drink warm.

- *Dosage:* 1 cup before bedtime

- *Caution:* Avoid if allergic to lavender

128. Ashwagandha (*Withania somnifera*)

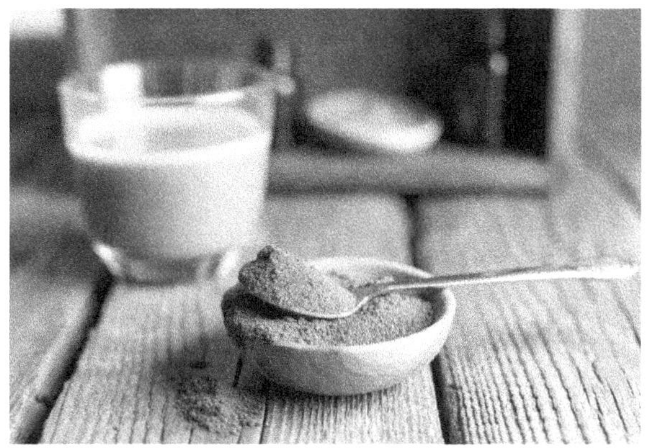

- *Part Used:* Root

- *Traditional Uses:* Stress, fatigue, anxiety

- *Preparation:*

1. Mix 1 teaspoon powdered root with warm water or milk.

2. Stir well and drink slowly.

- *Dosage:* Once daily, preferably evening

- *Caution:* Avoid in pregnancy

129. California Poppy (*Eschscholzia californica*)

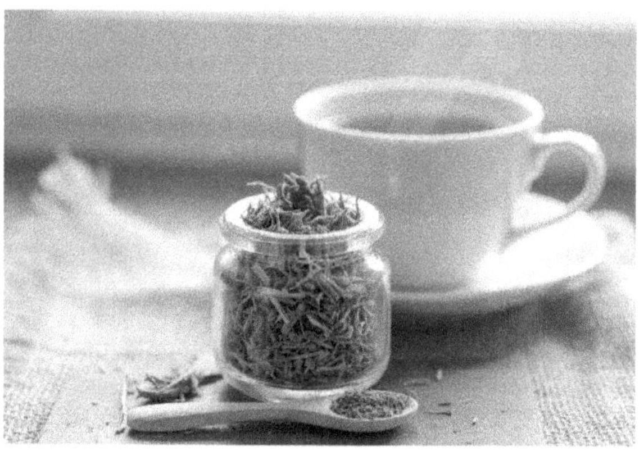

- *Part Used:* Aerial parts

- *Traditional Uses:* Insomnia, anxiety, pain relief

- *Preparation:*

1. Steep 1 teaspoon dried aerial parts in 1 cup boiling water.

2. Cover and steep for 10 minutes.

3. Strain and drink warm.

- *Dosage:* 1 cup before sleep

- *Caution:* Avoid in pregnancy

130. Magnolia Bark (*Magnolia officinalis*)

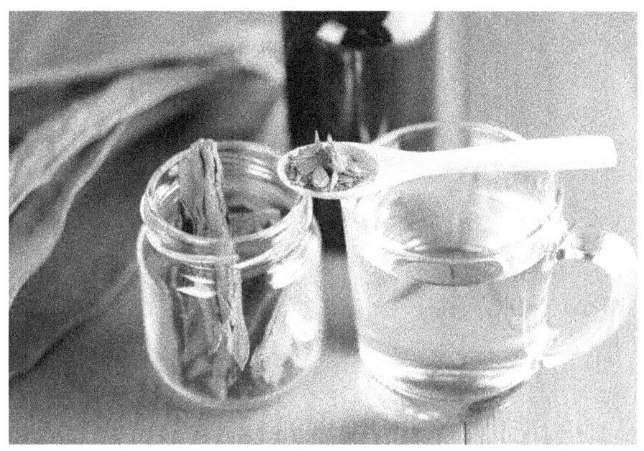

- *Part Used:* Bark

- *Traditional Uses:* Anxiety, stress, sleep aid

- *Preparation:*

1. Simmer 1 teaspoon dried bark in 1 cup water for 15 minutes.

2. Strain and drink warm.

- *Dosage:* 1 cup in the evening

- *Caution:* Avoid during pregnancy and breastfeeding

131. Lemon Verbena (*Aloysia citrodora*)

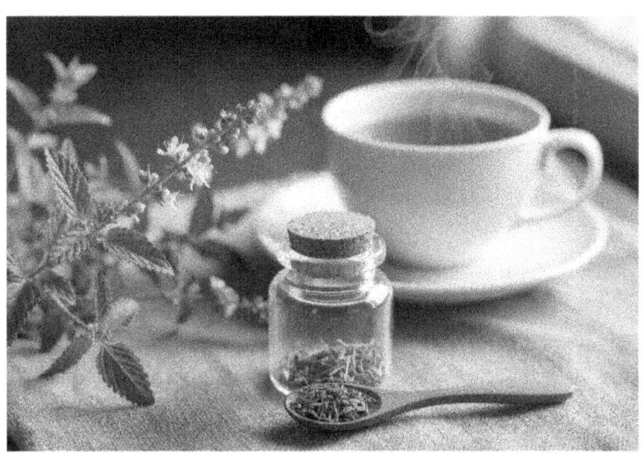

- *Part Used:* Leaves

- *Traditional Uses:* Stress, digestive aid, sleep

- *Preparation:*

1. Steep 1 tablespoon dried leaves in 1 cup boiling water.

2. Cover and steep for 10 minutes.

3. Strain and drink warm.

- *Dosage:* Up to 3 cups daily

- *Caution:* Avoid excessive use

132. Rose (*Rosa damascena*)

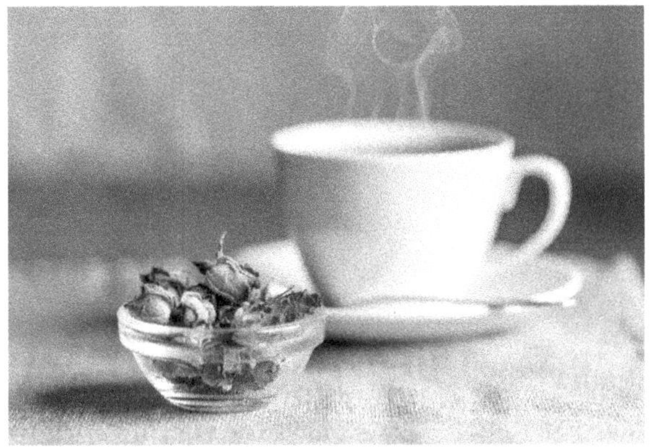

- *Part Used:* Flowers

- *Traditional Uses:* Mood support, mild sedative

- *Preparation:*

1. Steep 1 tablespoon dried rose petals in 1 cup hot water.

2. Cover and steep for 10 minutes.

3. Strain and drink warm.

- *Dosage:* 1–2 cups daily

- *Caution:* None known

133. St. John's Wort (*Hypericum perforatum*)

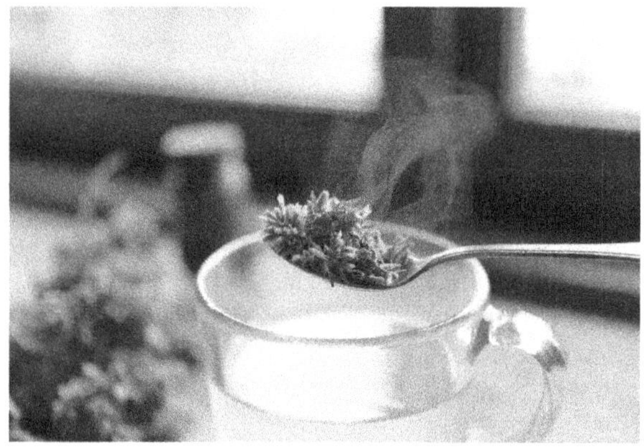

- ***Part Used:*** Flowers and leaves

- ***Traditional Uses:*** Depression, mood disorders

- ***Preparation:***

1. Steep 1 teaspoon dried herb in 1 cup boiling water.

2. Cover and steep for 10 minutes.

3. Strain and drink warm.

- ***Dosage:*** 1–3 cups daily

- ***Caution:*** Can interact with many medications

134. Ginkgo (*Ginkgo biloba*)

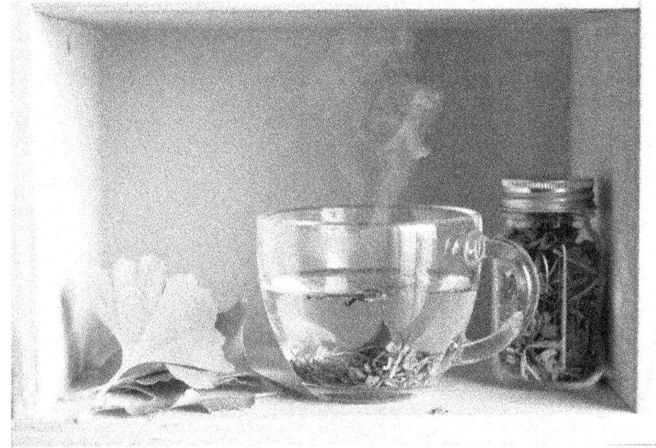

- *Part Used:* Leaves

- *Traditional Uses:* Memory, mental clarity, anxiety

- *Preparation:*

1. Steep 1 teaspoon dried leaves in 1 cup boiling water.

2. Cover and steep for 10 minutes.

3. Strain and drink.

- *Dosage:* 1–2 cups daily

- *Caution:* May increase bleeding risk

135. Lemon Balm (*Melissa officinalis*)

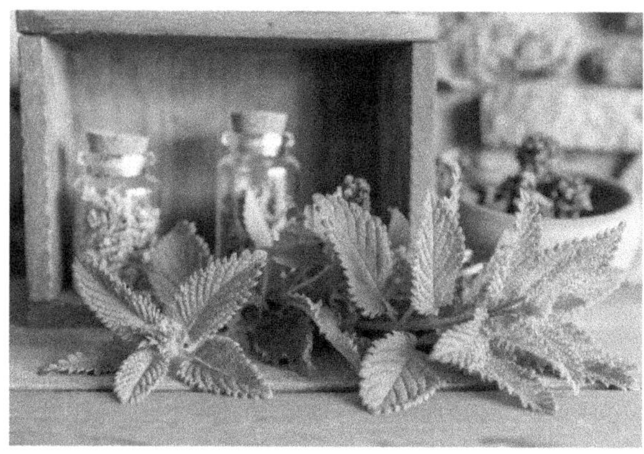

- *Part Used:* Leaves

- *Traditional Uses:* Stress, insomnia, digestive aid

- *Preparation:* (See Remedy 123)

- *Dosage:* (See Remedy 123)

- *Caution:* (See Remedy 123)

136. Kava Kava (*Piper methysticum*)

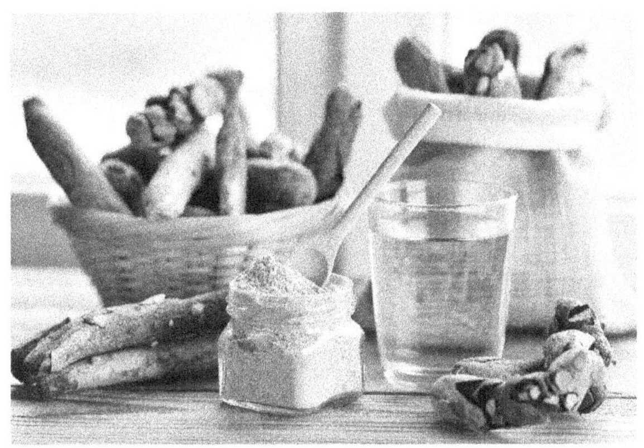

- ***Part Used:*** Root

- ***Traditional Uses:*** Anxiety, stress relief, muscle relaxation

- ***Preparation:***

1. Mix 1 teaspoon powdered root in warm water.

2. Knead or stir thoroughly.

3. Strain before drinking.

- ***Dosage:*** Short-term use only

- ***Caution:*** Risk of liver toxicity

137. Hops (*Humulus lupulus*)

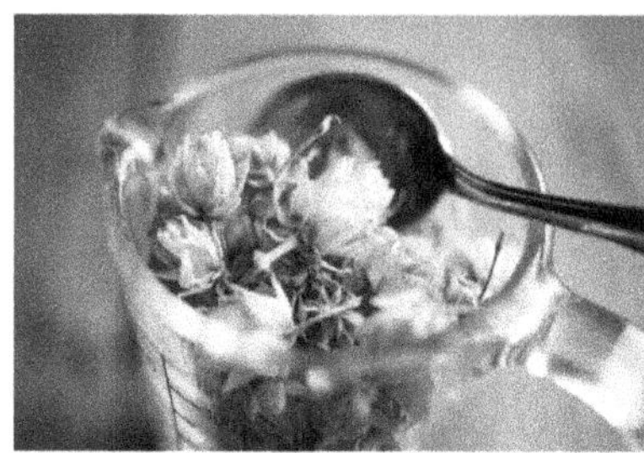

- *Part Used:* Flower cones

- *Traditional Uses:* Insomnia, anxiety, mild sedation

- *Preparation:*

1. Measure 1 tablespoon of dried hop flower cones.

2. Add to 1 cup of boiling water.

3. Cover and steep for 10 minutes.

4. Strain and drink warm.

- *Dosage:* 1 cup before bedtime

- *Caution:* May cause allergic reactions in sensitive individuals; avoid use during pregnancy and breastfeeding unless advised by a healthcare provider.

138. Chamomile (*Matricaria chamomilla*)

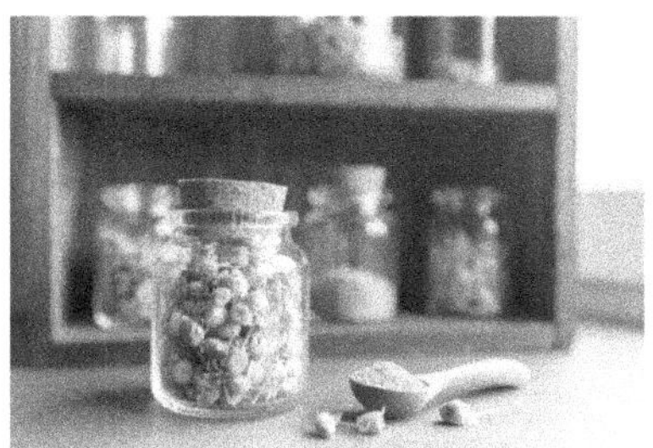

- **Part Used:** Flowers

- **Traditional Uses:** Sleep aid, anxiety relief, digestive support

- **Preparation:**

1. Use 1 tablespoon of dried chamomile flowers.

2. Pour 1 cup boiling water over the flowers.

3. Cover and steep for 10 minutes.

4. Strain and drink warm.

- **Dosage:** 1 cup before bedtime or up to 3 cups daily

- **Caution:** Possible allergic reactions especially if allergic to ragweed or related plants.

139. Lavender (*Lavandula angustifolia*)

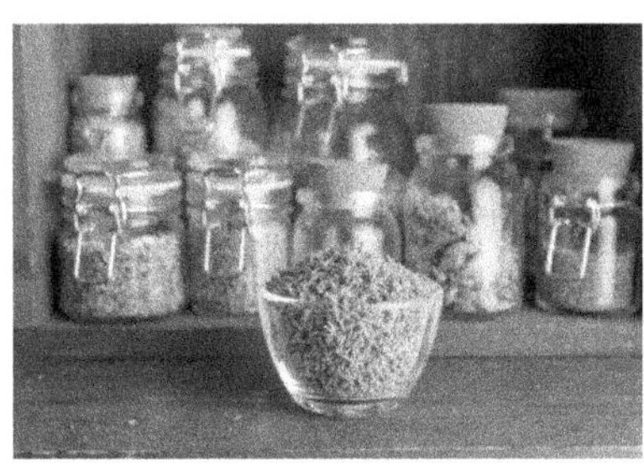

- **Part Used:** Flowers

- **Traditional Uses:** Anxiety reduction, insomnia, mood enhancement

- **Preparation:**

1. Place 1 tablespoon dried lavender flowers into a cup.

2. Pour 1 cup boiling water over the flowers.

3. Cover and steep for 10 minutes.

4. Strain and drink warm.

- **Dosage:** 1 cup before bedtime or as needed for relaxation

- **Caution:** Avoid if allergic to lavender; discontinue use if skin irritation occurs.

140. Skullcap (*Scutellaria lateriflora*)

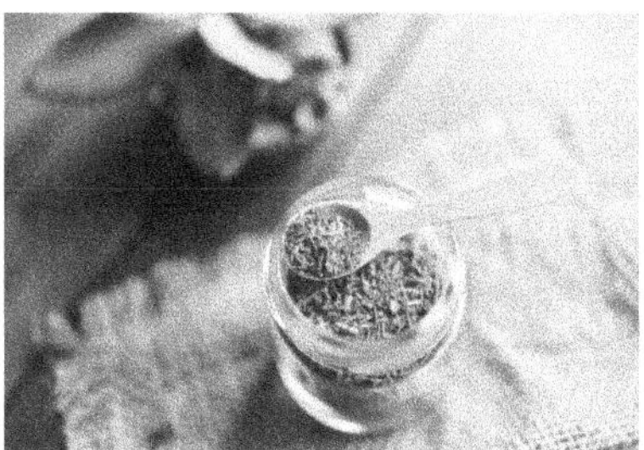

- **Part Used:** Aerial parts (leaves, stems, flowers)

- **Traditional Uses:** Nervous tension, insomnia, mild sedative

- **Preparation:**

1. Measure 1 teaspoon dried skullcap herb.

2. Pour 1 cup boiling water over the herb.

3. Cover and steep for 10 minutes.

4. Strain and drink warm.

- **Dosage:** 1–2 cups daily, preferably in the evening

- **Caution:** Avoid prolonged use; consult a healthcare professional if pregnant or nursing.

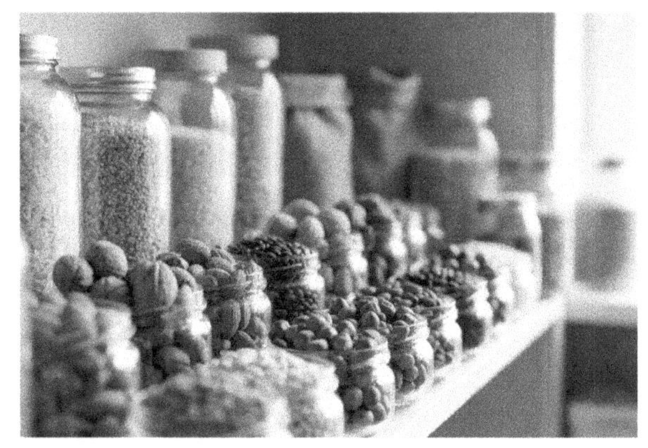

SECTION III: SEEDS, NUTS & GRAINS
(Remedies 141–200)

Digestive, Appetite & Weight-support Seeds (141–160)

141. Fennel (*Foeniculum vulgare*)

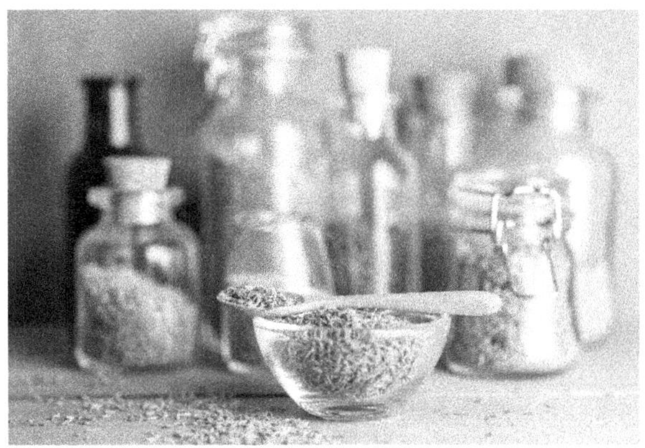

- *Part Used:* Seeds

- *Traditional Uses:* Digestive aid, bloating, appetite stimulant

- *Preparation:*

1. Lightly crush 1 teaspoon of fennel seeds.

2. Add to 1 cup boiling water.

3. Cover and steep for 10 minutes.

4. Strain and drink warm.

- *Dosage:* 1–2 cups daily after meals

- *Caution:* Avoid high doses during pregnancy

142. Cumin (*Cuminum cyminum*)

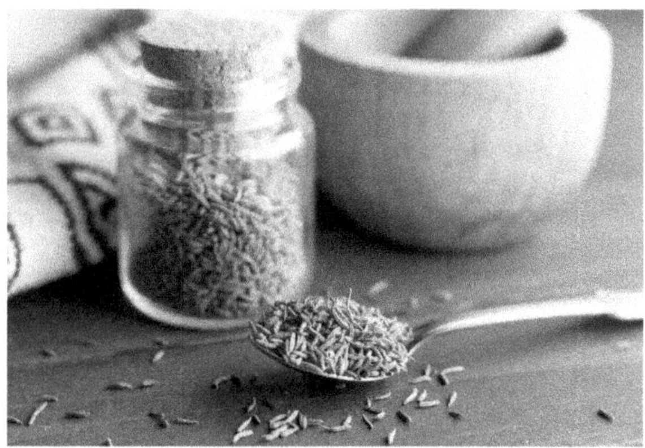

- ***Part Used:*** Seeds

- ***Traditional Uses:*** Digestion, gas relief, appetite stimulation

- ***Preparation:***

1. Roast 1 teaspoon cumin seeds lightly (optional).

2. Crush seeds gently.

3. Steep in 1 cup boiling water for 10 minutes.

4. Strain and drink warm.

- ***Dosage:*** 1–2 cups daily

- ***Caution:*** Use moderately during pregnancy

143. Coriander (*Coriandrum sativum*)

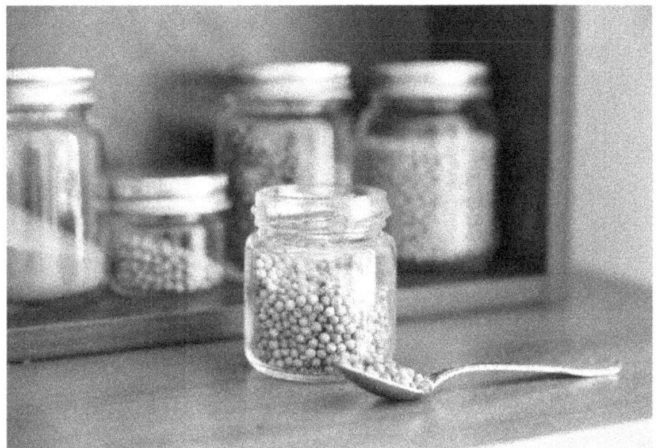

- *Part Used:* Seeds

- *Traditional Uses:* Digestion, detoxification, appetite support

- *Preparation:*

1. Lightly crush 1 teaspoon coriander seeds.

2. Add to 1 cup boiling water.

3. Cover and steep for 10 minutes.

4. Strain and drink warm.

- *Dosage:* 1–2 cups daily

- *Caution:* None known in normal doses

144. Caraway (*Carum carvi*)

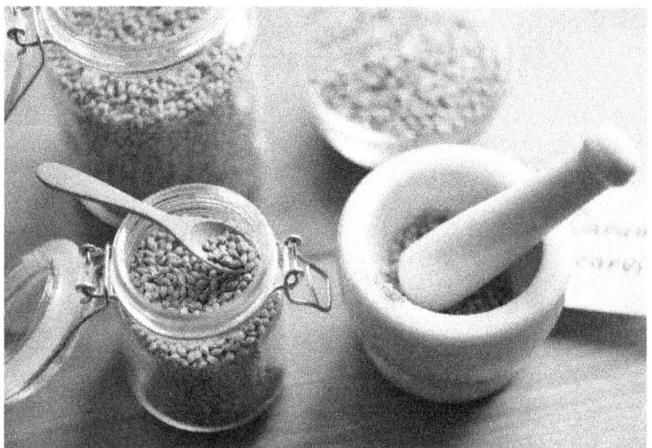

- ***Part Used:*** Seeds

- ***Traditional Uses:*** Digestive discomfort, bloating, appetite

- ***Preparation:***

1. Crush 1 teaspoon caraway seeds lightly.

2. Steep in 1 cup boiling water for 10 minutes.

3. Strain and drink warm.

- ***Dosage:*** 1–2 cups daily after meals

- ***Caution:*** Avoid high doses during pregnancy

145. Cardamom (*Elettaria cardamomum*)

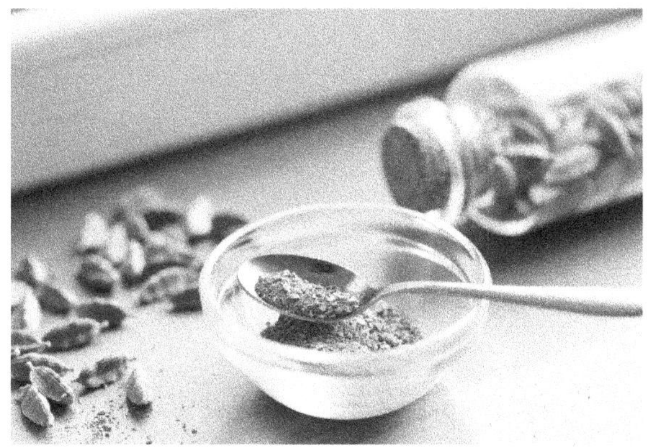

- *Part Used:* Seeds

- *Traditional Uses:* Digestion, nausea, appetite

- *Preparation:*

1. Lightly crush 1 teaspoon cardamom seeds.

2. Add to 1 cup boiling water.

3. Cover and steep for 10 minutes.

4. Strain and drink warm.

- *Dosage:* 1 cup daily

- *Caution:* Generally safe, avoid excessive amounts

146. Psyllium (*Plantago ovata*)

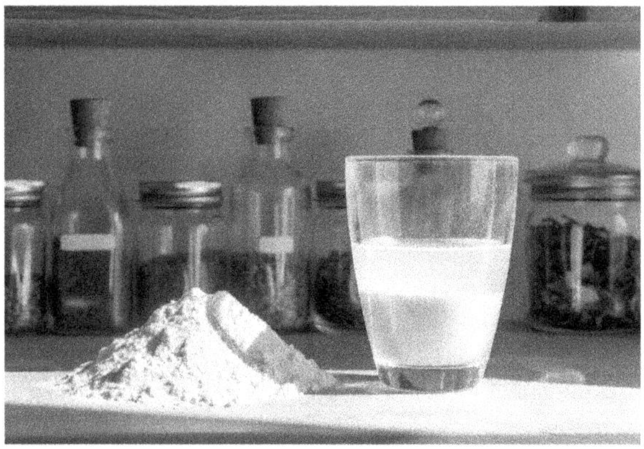

- *Part Used:* Seeds/husk

- *Traditional Uses:* Constipation, digestive cleansing, weight control

- *Preparation:*

1. Mix 1 teaspoon psyllium husk or seeds in 1 glass (250 ml) of water.

2. Stir well and drink immediately.

3. Follow with an additional glass of water.

- *Dosage:* 1–2 times daily

- *Caution:* Drink plenty of water to avoid choking

147. Flaxseed (*Linum usitatissimum*)

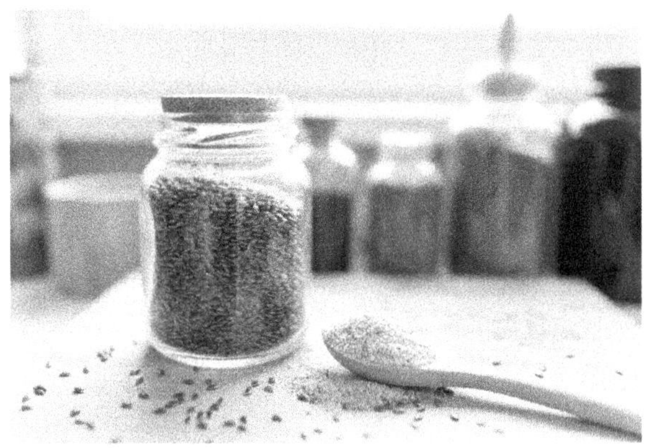

- *Part Used:* Seeds

- *Traditional Uses:* Digestion, constipation, weight management

- *Preparation:*

1. Grind 1 tablespoon flaxseeds.

2. Mix with water, juice, or add to smoothies.

3. Consume immediately.

- *Dosage:* 1 tablespoon daily

- *Caution:* Increase fiber intake gradually

148. Pumpkin Seeds (*Cucurbita pepo*)

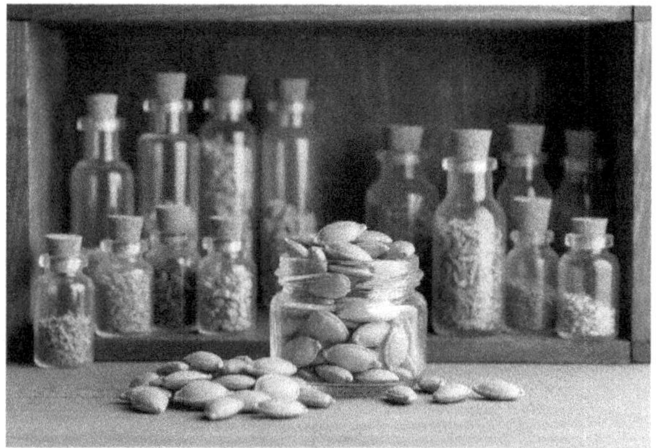

- **Part Used:** Seeds

- **Traditional Uses:** Appetite suppressant, digestion, prostate health

- **Preparation:**

1. Consume raw or roasted seeds.

2. Alternatively, grind seeds and add to food or drinks.

- **Dosage:** 1–2 tablespoons daily

- **Caution:** Allergies possible

149. Sesame Seeds (*Sesamum indicum*)

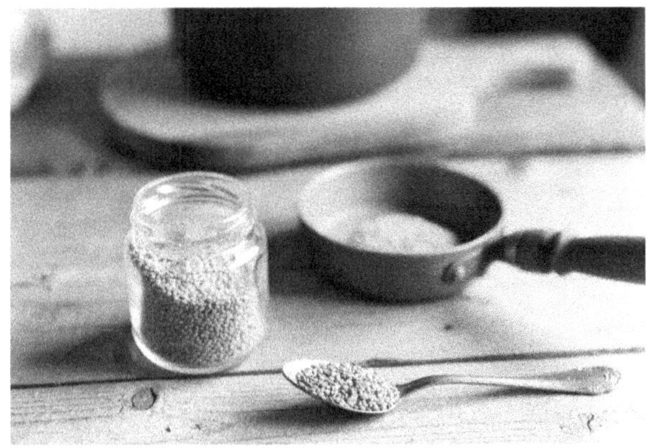

- *Part Used:* Seeds

- *Traditional Uses:* Digestion, metabolism support, appetite

- *Preparation:*

1. Toast 1 tablespoon sesame seeds lightly.

2. Grind and mix with honey or water.

3. Consume directly or add to food.

- *Dosage:* 1 tablespoon daily

- *Caution:* Allergies possible

150. Nigella Seed (Black Seed) (*Nigella sativa*)

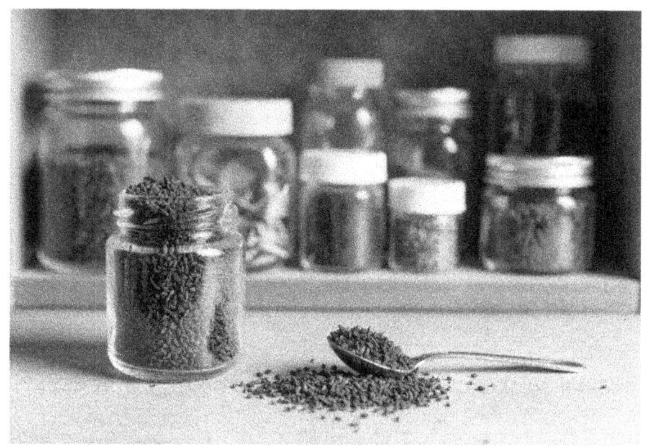

- *Part Used:* Seeds

- *Traditional Uses:* Digestion, appetite, immunity

- *Preparation:*

1. Crush 1 teaspoon seeds.

2. Mix with honey or take with warm water.

- *Dosage:* ½ to 1 teaspoon daily

- *Caution:* Avoid during pregnancy

151. Aniseed (*Pimpinella anisum*)

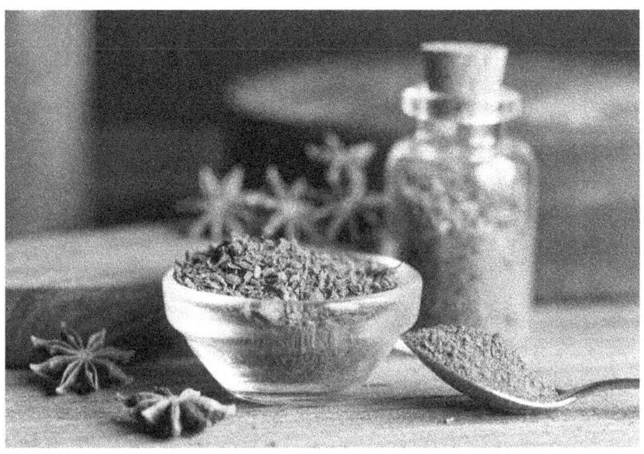

- *Part Used:* Seeds

- *Traditional Uses:* Digestion, gas relief, appetite stimulant

- *Preparation:*

1. Lightly crush 1 teaspoon aniseed.

2. Steep in 1 cup boiling water for 10 minutes.

3. Strain and drink warm.

- *Dosage:* 1–2 cups daily

- *Caution:* Avoid if allergic to plants in the carrot family

152. Celery Seeds (*Apium graveolens*)

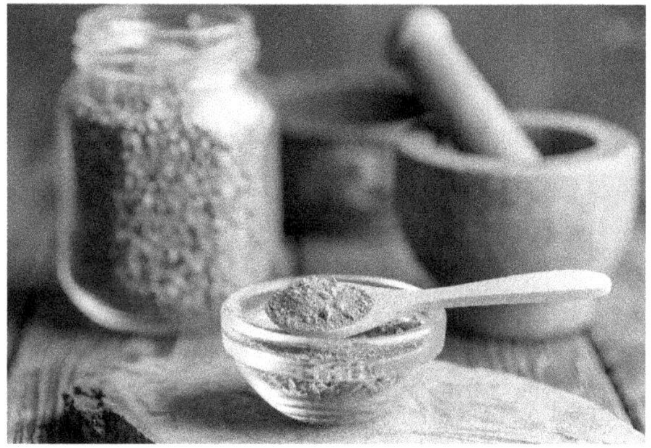

- *Part Used:* Seeds

- *Traditional Uses:* Digestion, appetite, diuretic

- *Preparation:*

1. Crush 1 teaspoon celery seeds.

2. Add to 1 cup boiling water.

3. Cover and steep for 10 minutes.

4. Strain and drink warm.

- *Dosage:* 1 cup daily

- *Caution:* Avoid in pregnancy and allergies

153. Carob Seeds (*Ceratonia siliqua*)

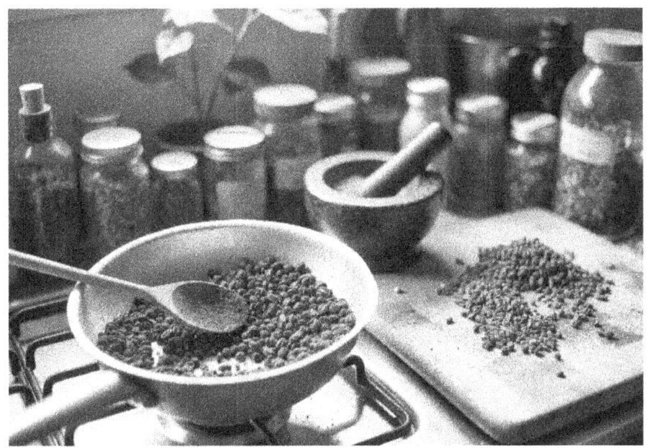

- *Part Used:* Seeds

- *Traditional Uses:* Digestive health, appetite

- *Preparation:*

1. Roast and grind seeds.

2. Add powder to hot water or milk.

3. Stir well and drink warm.

- *Dosage:* 1 cup daily

- *Caution:* Generally safe

154. Mustard Seeds (*Brassica nigra*)

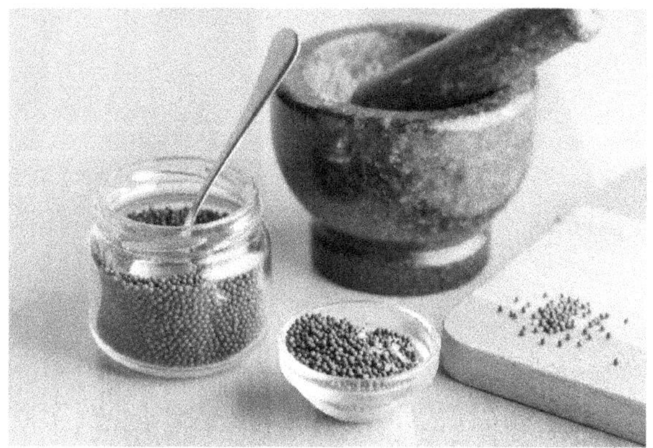

- ***Part Used:*** Seeds

- ***Traditional Uses:*** Digestion, metabolism booster

- ***Preparation:***

1. Lightly crush ½ teaspoon mustard seeds.

2. Add to hot water or food.

- ***Dosage:*** Small amounts due to potency

- ***Caution:*** Avoid in large doses; may irritate mucous membranes

155. Celery Seeds (*Apium graveolens*)

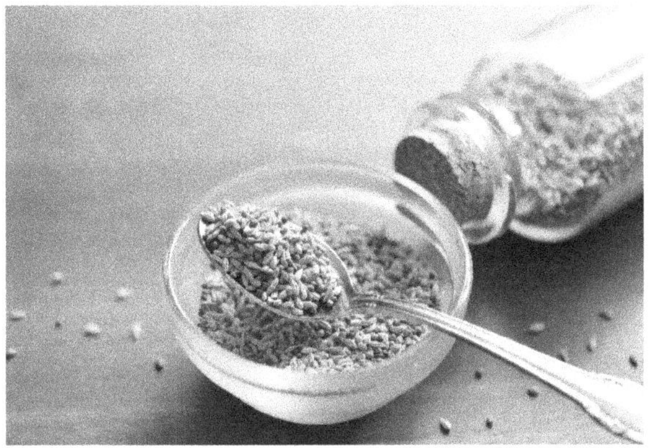

- *Part Used:* Seeds

- *Traditional Uses:* Digestion, appetite stimulant, mild diuretic

- *Preparation:*

1. Lightly crush 1 teaspoon of celery seeds.

2. Add to 1 cup boiling water.

3. Cover and steep for 10 minutes.

4. Strain and drink warm.

- *Dosage:* 1 cup daily after meals

- *Caution:* Avoid during pregnancy and if allergic to celery family plants

156. Fennel Seeds (*Foeniculum vulgare*)

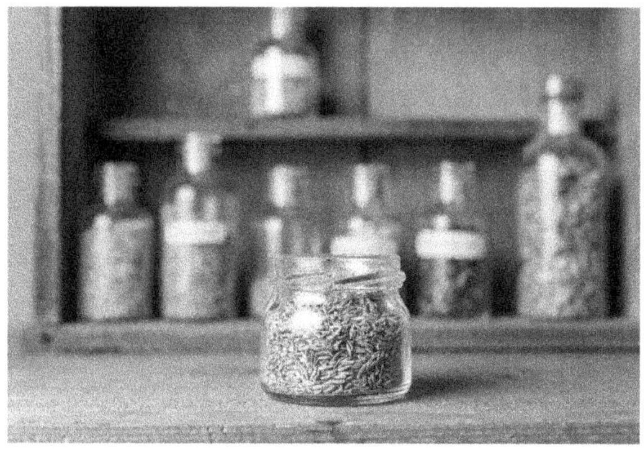

- *Part Used:* Seeds

- *Traditional Uses:* Digestive aid, bloating relief, appetite support

- *Preparation:*

1. Lightly crush 1 teaspoon of fennel seeds.

2. Add to 1 cup boiling water.

3. Cover and steep for 10 minutes.

4. Strain and drink warm.

- *Dosage:* 1–2 cups daily after meals

- *Caution:* Avoid high doses during pregnancy

157. Coriander Seeds (*Coriandrum sativum*)

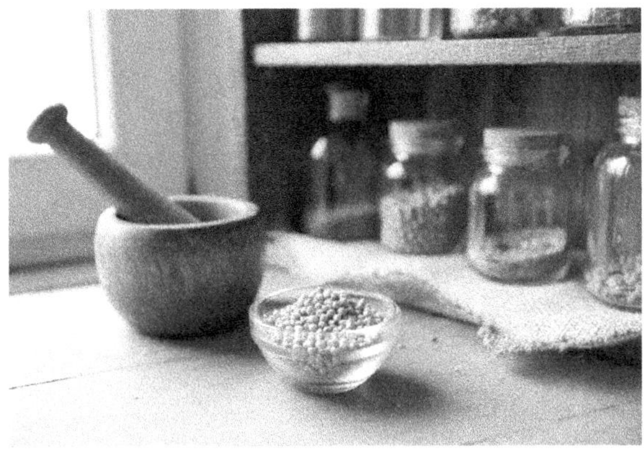

- *Part Used:* Seeds

- *Traditional Uses:* Digestion, detoxification, appetite enhancement

- *Preparation:*

1. Lightly crush 1 teaspoon coriander seeds.

2. Add to 1 cup boiling water.

3. Cover and steep for 10 minutes.

4. Strain and drink warm.

- *Dosage:* 1–2 cups daily

- *Caution:* Generally safe in normal amounts

158. Cumin Seeds (*Cuminum cyminum*)

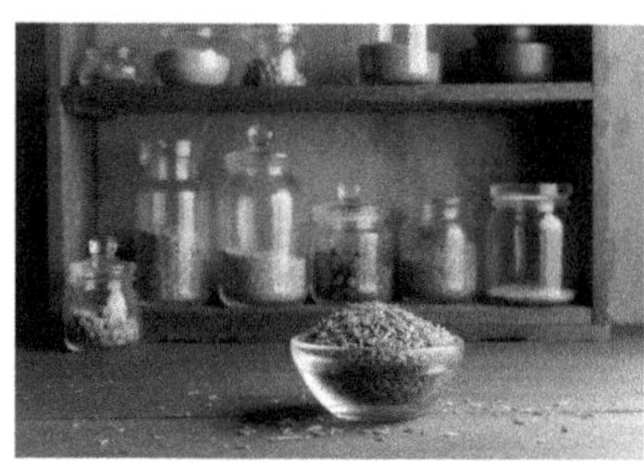

- *Part Used:* Seeds

- *Traditional Uses:* Digestion, gas relief, appetite stimulation

- *Preparation:*

1. Roast 1 teaspoon cumin seeds lightly (optional).

2. Crush gently.

3. Add to 1 cup boiling water.

4. Cover and steep for 10 minutes.

5. Strain and drink warm.

- *Dosage:* 1–2 cups daily

- *Caution:* Use moderately during pregnancy

159. Pumpkin Seeds (*Cucurbita pepo*)

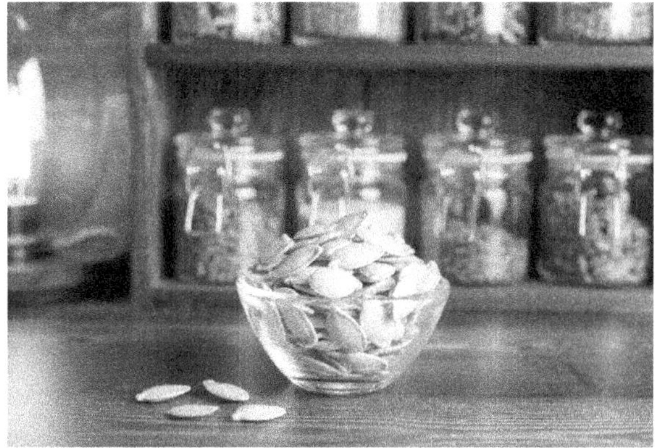

- *Part Used:* Seeds

- *Traditional Uses:* Appetite suppressant, digestion aid, prostate health

- *Preparation:*

1. Consume raw or lightly roasted seeds as a snack.

2. Alternatively, grind seeds and add to food or drinks.

- *Dosage:* 1–2 tablespoons daily

- *Caution:* Possible allergic reactions in some individuals

160. Sesame Seeds (*Sesamum indicum*)

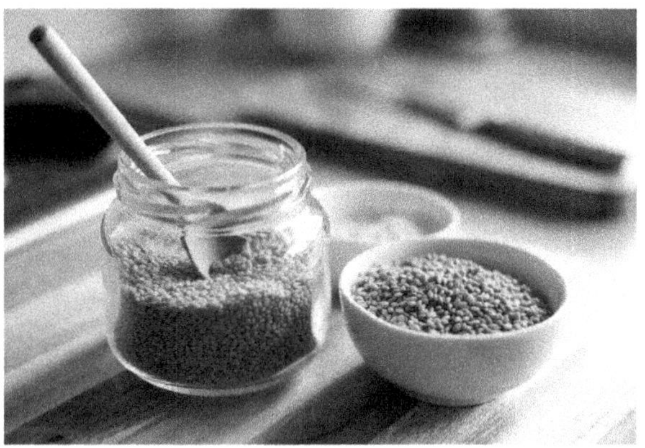

- *Part Used:* Seeds

- *Traditional Uses:* Digestive health, metabolism support, appetite

- *Preparation:*

1. Lightly toast 1 tablespoon sesame seeds.

2. Grind seeds into a powder.

3. Mix powder with honey or warm water.

4. Consume directly or add to meals.

- *Dosage:* 1 tablespoon daily

- *Caution:* Possible allergies; avoid excessive intake

Hormonal, Fertility & Reproductive Health Seeds (161–180)

161. Fenugreek (*Trigonella foenum-graecum*)

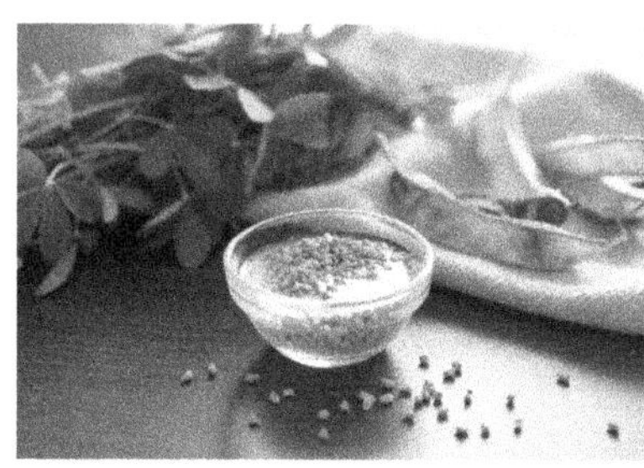

- *Part Used:* Seeds

- *Traditional Uses:* Hormonal balance, lactation support, fertility

- *Preparation:*

1. Soak 1 tablespoon of fenugreek seeds in water overnight.

2. Strain seeds and chew or prepare as tea by boiling soaked seeds in 1 cup water for 10 minutes.

3. Strain and drink warm.

- *Dosage:* 1 cup daily

- *Caution:* May cause body odor; avoid during pregnancy without medical advice

162. Pumpkin Seeds (*Cucurbita pepo*)

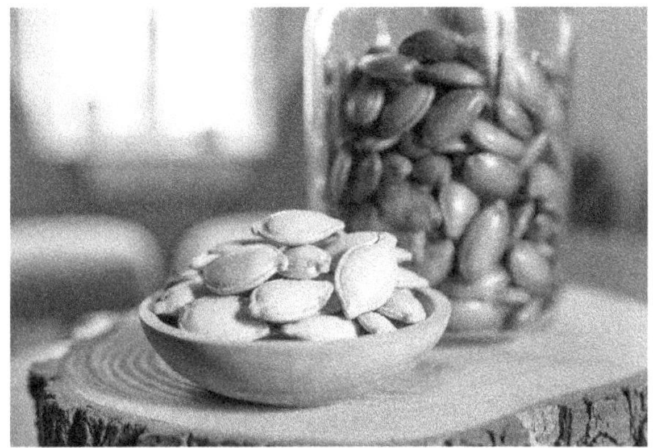

- *Part Used:* Seeds

- *Traditional Uses:* Prostate health, hormonal balance, fertility

- *Preparation:*

1. Consume raw or roasted seeds as a snack.

2. Alternatively, grind seeds and add to food or drinks.

- *Dosage:* 1–2 tablespoons daily

- *Caution:* Allergies possible

163. Sesame Seeds (*Sesamum indicum*)

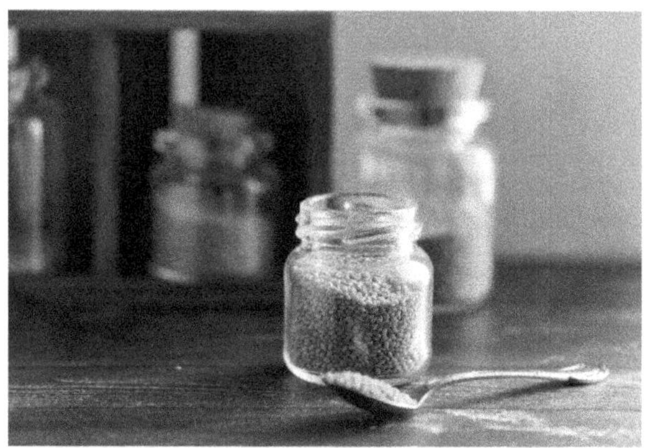

- *Part Used:* Seeds

- *Traditional Uses:* Hormone regulation, fertility, menstrual health

- *Preparation:*

1. Lightly toast 1 tablespoon sesame seeds.

2. Grind into powder.

3. Mix with honey or warm water and consume.

- *Dosage:* 1 tablespoon daily

- *Caution:* Possible allergies; avoid excess intake

164. Black Cohosh (*Actaea racemosa*)

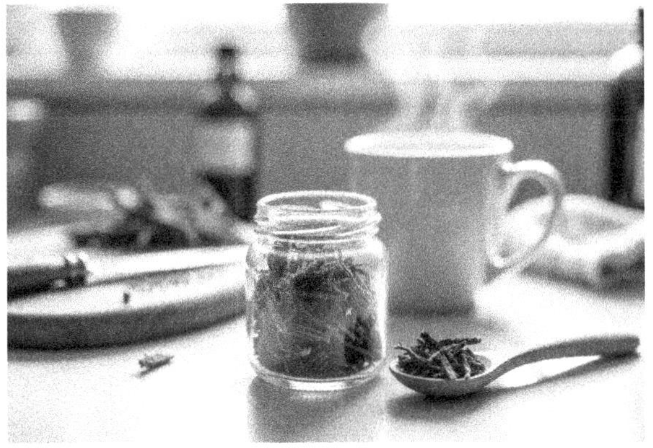

- *Part Used:* Root

- *Traditional Uses:* Menopause symptoms, menstrual cramps

- *Preparation:*

1. Add 1 teaspoon dried root to 1 cup boiling water.

2. Steep for 10–15 minutes.

3. Strain and drink warm.

- *Dosage:* 1 cup daily

- *Caution:* Not recommended during pregnancy or breastfeeding; possible liver toxicity with long-term use

165. Red Clover (*Trifolium pratense*)

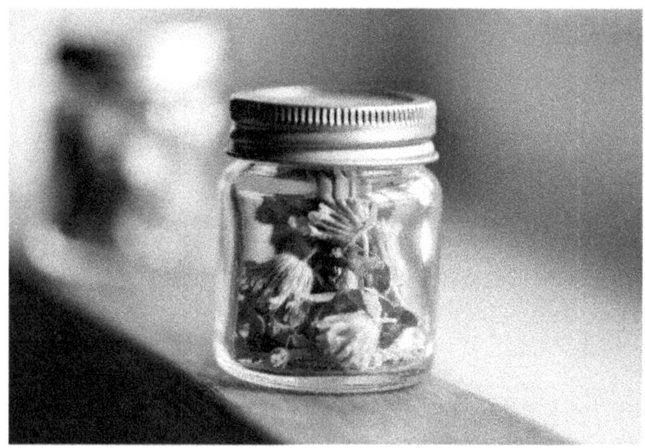

- *Part Used:* Flowers

- *Traditional Uses:* Menopause support, hormonal balance

- *Preparation:*

1. Use 1 tablespoon dried flowers.

2. Pour boiling water (1 cup) over flowers.

3. Cover and steep for 10 minutes.

4. Strain and drink warm.

- *Dosage:* 1–2 cups daily

- *Caution:* Avoid if prone to hormone-sensitive conditions

166. Flaxseed (*Linum usitatissimum*)

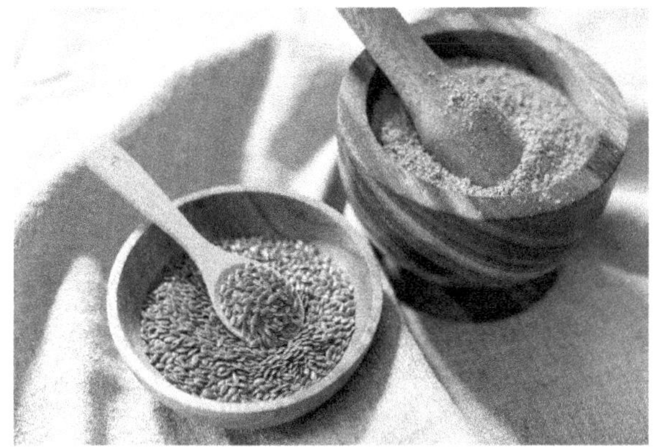

- *Part Used:* Seeds

- *Traditional Uses:* Hormonal balance, fertility support, menstrual health

- *Preparation:*

1. Grind 1 tablespoon flaxseeds.

2. Mix with water, juice, or add to smoothies.

- *Dosage:* 1 tablespoon daily

- *Caution:* Increase fiber gradually; avoid if prone to hormone-sensitive cancers

167. Saw Palmetto (*Serenoa repens*)

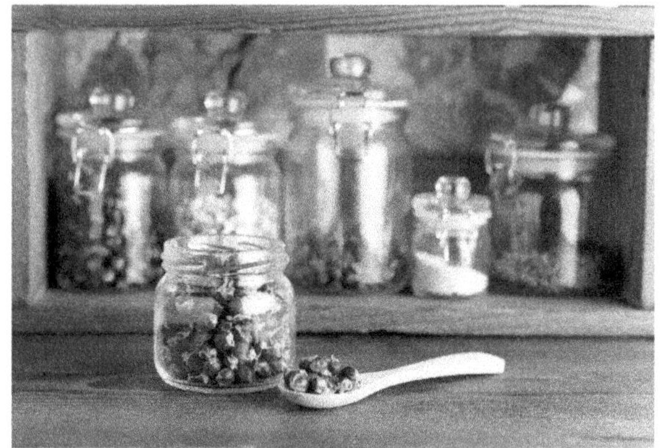

- ***Part Used:*** Fruit/berries

- ***Traditional Uses:*** Prostate health, hormone regulation

- ***Preparation:***

1. Use dried berries; crush 1 teaspoon.

2. Steep in 1 cup boiling water for 10–15 minutes.

3. Strain and drink.

- ***Dosage:*** 1 cup daily

- ***Caution:*** Consult doctor if on hormone therapy or blood thinners

168. Maca (*Lepidium meyenii*)

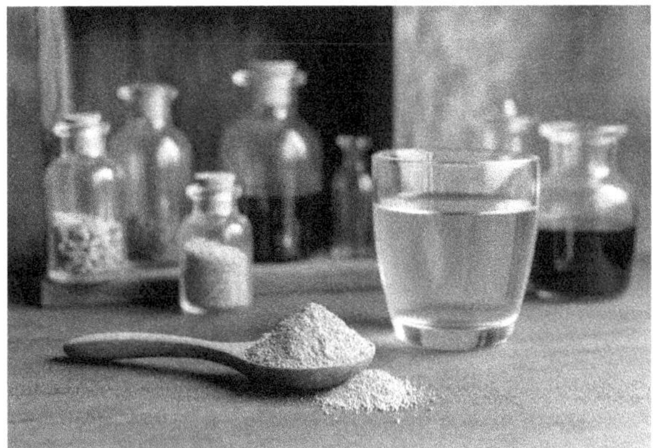

- ***Part Used:*** Root

- ***Traditional Uses:*** Energy, fertility, hormonal balance

- ***Preparation:***

1. Add 1 teaspoon maca powder to warm water, milk, or smoothies.

2. Stir well and consume.

- ***Dosage:*** 1 teaspoon daily

- ***Caution:*** Avoid if thyroid problems; monitor hormonal effects

169. Evening Primrose (*Oenothera biennis*)

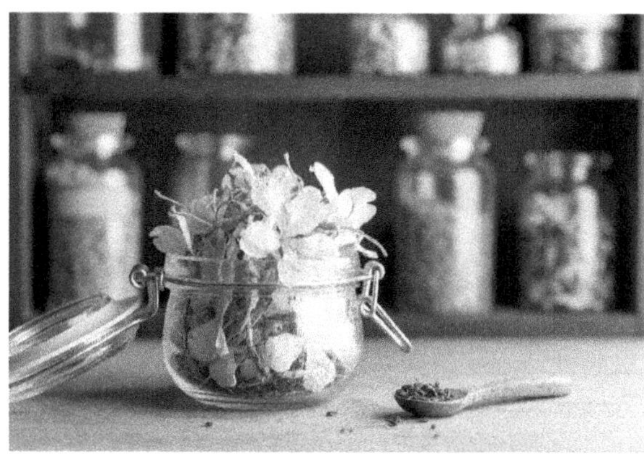

- *Part Used:* Seeds

- *Traditional Uses:* PMS, menopause symptoms, skin health

- *Preparation:*

1. Take oil capsules or consume 1 teaspoon of evening primrose oil.

- *Dosage:* 1 teaspoon daily or per capsule instructions

- *Caution:* May interact with blood thinners; consult doctor

170. Chasteberry (*Vitex agnus-castus*)

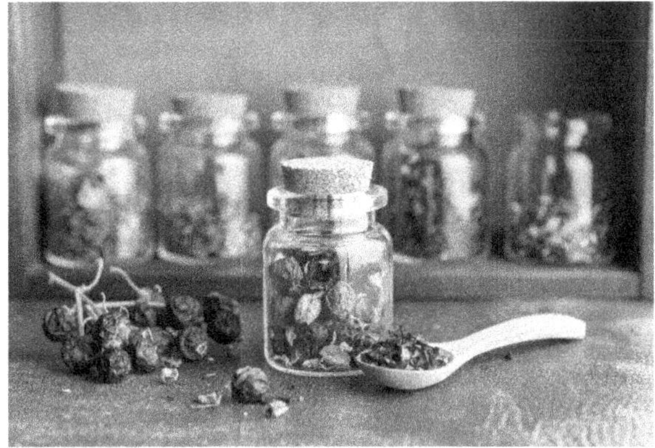

- ***Part Used:*** Fruit/berries

- ***Traditional Uses:*** PMS, menstrual irregularities, hormonal balance

- ***Preparation:***

1. Use dried berries; crush 1 teaspoon.

2. Steep in 1 cup boiling water for 10–15 minutes.

3. Strain and drink warm.

- ***Dosage:*** 1 cup daily

- ***Caution:*** Avoid during pregnancy; may interfere with hormone therapies

171. Tribulus (*Tribulus terrestris*)

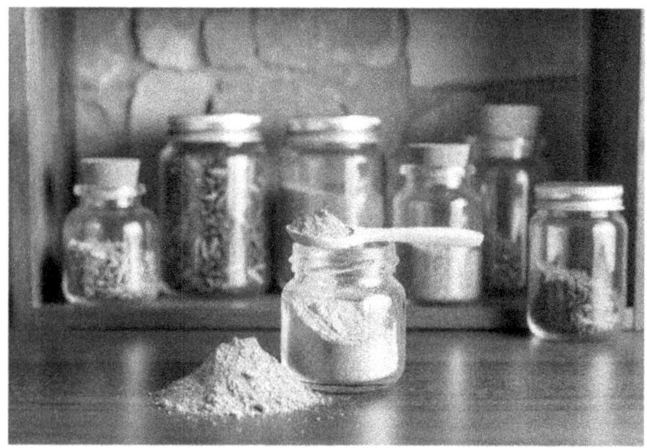

- *Part Used:* Fruit

- *Traditional Uses:* Fertility, libido enhancement, hormonal support

- *Preparation:*

1. Use dried fruit powder or extract as per instructions.

2. For tea, steep 1 teaspoon dried fruit in 1 cup boiling water for 10 minutes.

3. Strain and drink.

- *Dosage:* 1 cup daily

- *Caution:* Monitor hormone-sensitive conditions

172. Dong Quai (*Angelica sinensis*)

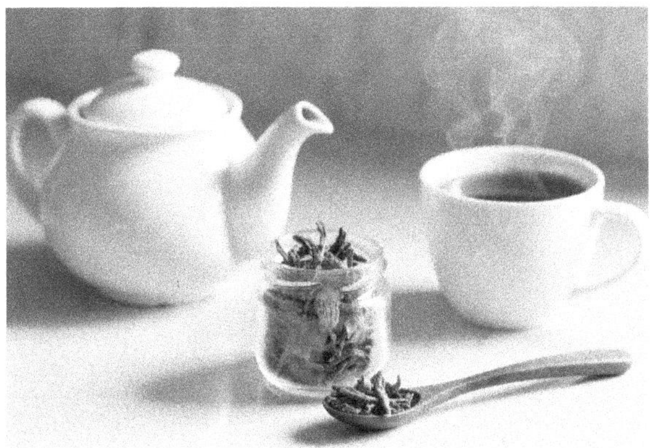

- *Part Used:* Root

- *Traditional Uses:* Menstrual cramps, menopausal symptoms, hormonal balance

- *Preparation:*

1. Add 1 teaspoon dried root to 1 cup boiling water.

2. Simmer gently for 15 minutes.

3. Strain and drink warm.

- *Dosage:* 1 cup daily

- *Caution:* Avoid during pregnancy; may increase photosensitivity

173. Ashwagandha (*Withania somnifera*)

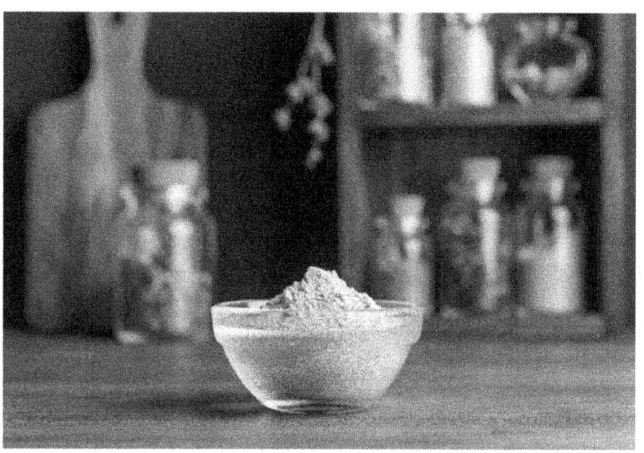

- *Part Used:* Root

- *Traditional Uses:* Stress relief, hormonal balance, fertility support

- *Preparation:*

1. Mix 1 teaspoon powdered root in warm water or milk.

2. Stir until dissolved.

- *Dosage:* Once daily, preferably at night

- *Caution:* Avoid during pregnancy

174. Horny Goat Weed (*Epimedium spp.*)

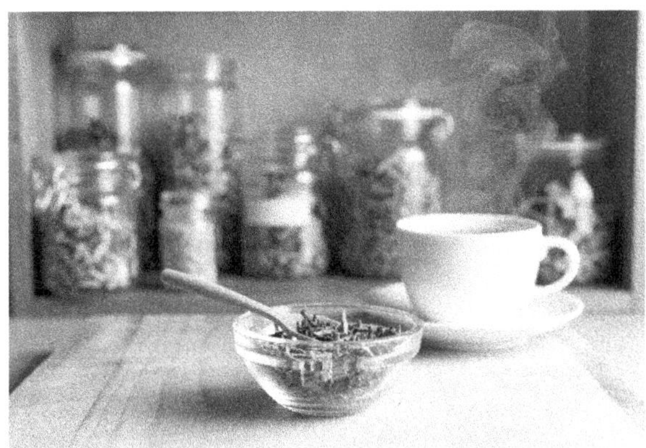

- *Part Used:* Leaves

- *Traditional Uses:* Libido enhancement, hormonal support

- *Preparation:*

1. Add 1 teaspoon dried leaves to 1 cup boiling water.

2. Steep for 10 minutes.

3. Strain and drink warm.

- *Dosage:* 1 cup daily

- *Caution:* Avoid high doses; consult doctor if on medications

175. Sarsaparilla (*Smilax spp.*)

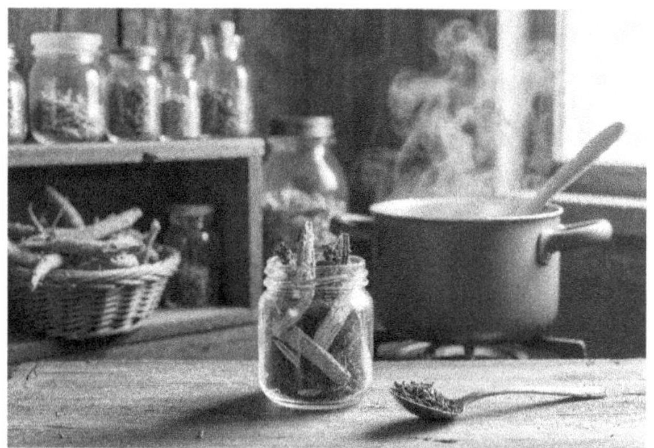

- *Part Used:* Root

- *Traditional Uses:* Hormonal balance, skin health, libido

- *Preparation:*

1. Boil 1 tablespoon dried root in 2 cups water for 15 minutes.

2. Strain and drink warm.

- *Dosage:* 1 cup daily

- *Caution:* Avoid excess use

176. Nettle Seed (*Urtica dioica*)

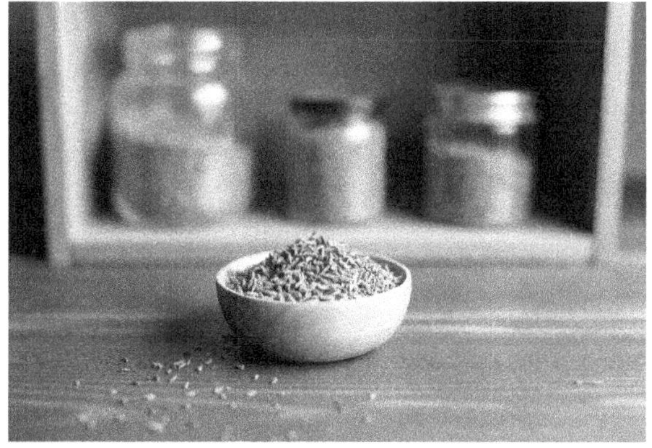

- *Part Used:* Seeds

- *Traditional Uses:* Fertility, hormone support

- *Preparation:*

1. Use 1 teaspoon dried seeds.

2. Add to 1 cup boiling water.

3. Steep for 10 minutes.

4. Strain and drink warm.

- *Dosage:* 1 cup daily

- *Caution:* Avoid allergy; consult doctor if pregnant

177. Black Seed (*Nigella sativa*)

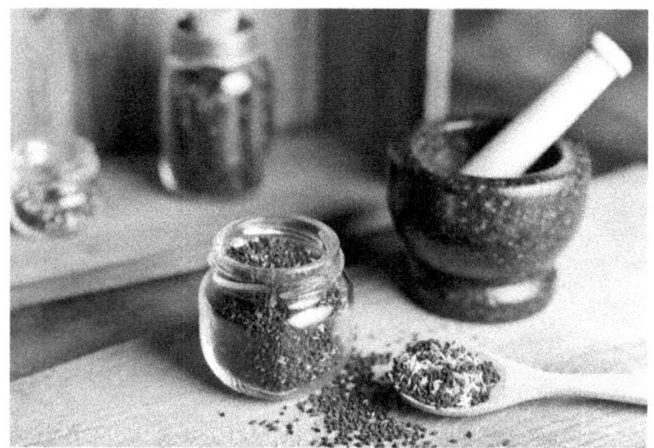

- *Part Used:* Seeds

- *Traditional Uses:* Hormonal balance, immunity, fertility

- *Preparation:*

1. Crush ½ to 1 teaspoon seeds.

2. Mix with honey or warm water.

- *Dosage:* ½ to 1 teaspoon daily

- *Caution:* Avoid during pregnancy

178. Pumpkin Seed (*Cucurbita pepo*)

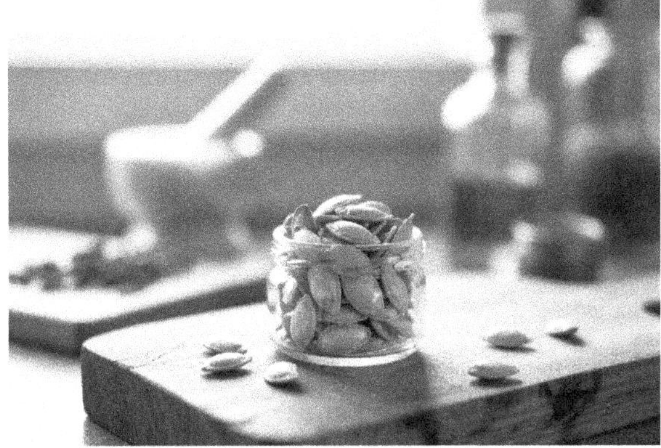

- *Part Used:* Seeds

- *Traditional Uses:* Hormonal balance, prostate health

- *Preparation:*

1. Consume raw or roasted seeds as snack.

2. Or grind seeds and add to food or drinks.

- *Dosage:* 1–2 tablespoons daily

- *Caution:* Allergies possible

179. Shatavari (*Asparagus racemosus*)

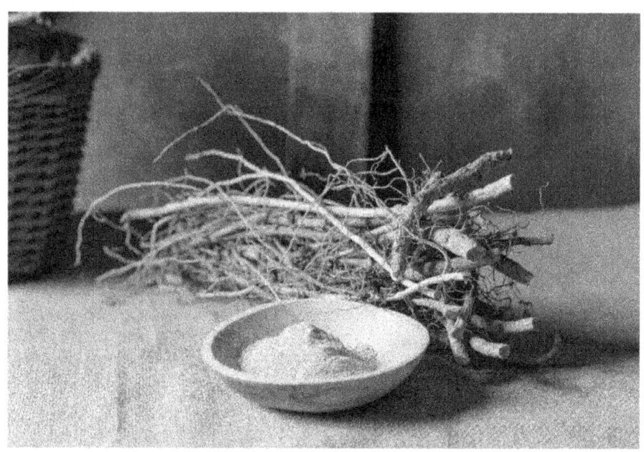

- *Part Used:* Root

- *Traditional Uses:* Female reproductive health, fertility, hormonal balance

- *Preparation:*

1. Add 1 teaspoon powdered root to warm water or milk.

2. Stir well and drink.

- *Dosage:* 1 cup daily

- *Caution:* Avoid if allergic to asparagus family

180. Mucuna (*Mucuna pruriens*)

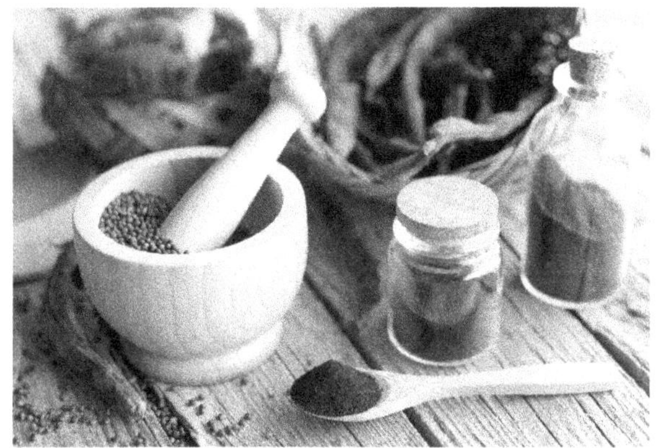

- ***Part Used:*** Seeds

- ***Traditional Uses:*** Fertility, libido, hormone support

- ***Preparation:***

1. Roast and grind seeds into powder.

2. Mix 1 teaspoon powder with warm water or milk.

3. Stir and drink.

- ***Dosage:*** 1 cup daily

- ***Caution:*** Avoid excess; consult doctor if on medication

Heart, Blood Sugar & Cholesterol-support Seeds (181–200)

181. Flaxseed (*Linum usitatissimum*)

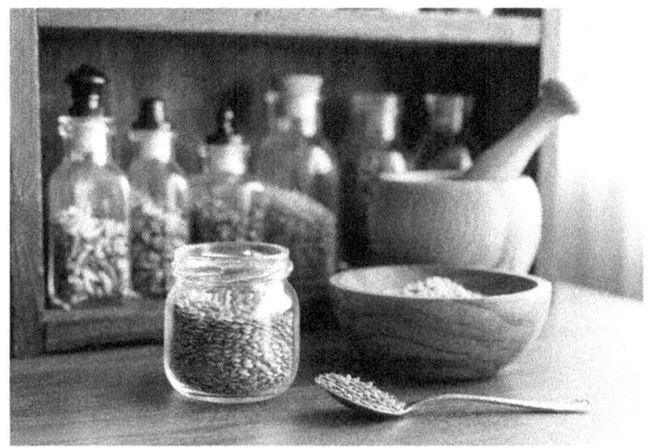

- *Part Used:* Seeds

- *Traditional Uses:* Cholesterol reduction, heart health, blood sugar control

- *Preparation:*

1. Grind 1 tablespoon flaxseeds fresh before use.

2. Mix with water, juice, or add to smoothies.

- *Dosage:* 1 tablespoon daily

- *Caution:* Increase fiber intake gradually; avoid if prone to hormone-sensitive cancers.

182. Fenugreek (*Trigonella foenum-graecum*)

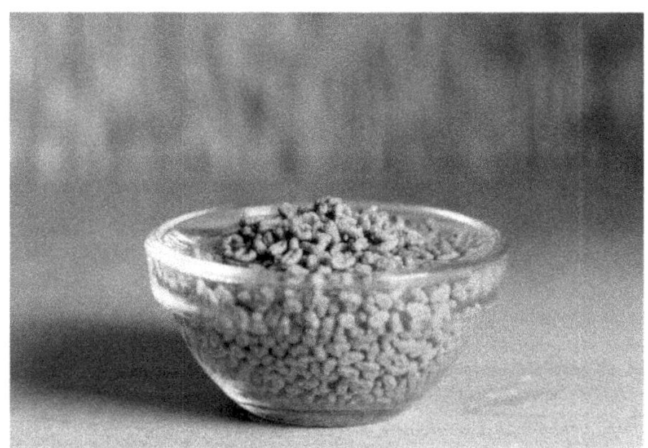

- *Part Used:* Seeds

- *Traditional Uses:* Blood sugar regulation, cholesterol management

- *Preparation:*

1. Soak 1 tablespoon seeds overnight in water.

2. Drink the water and chew seeds or boil soaked seeds in 1 cup water for 10 minutes, then strain and drink.

- *Dosage:* 1 cup daily

- *Caution:* May cause body odor; avoid in pregnancy without medical advice.

183. Pumpkin Seeds (*Cucurbita pepo*)

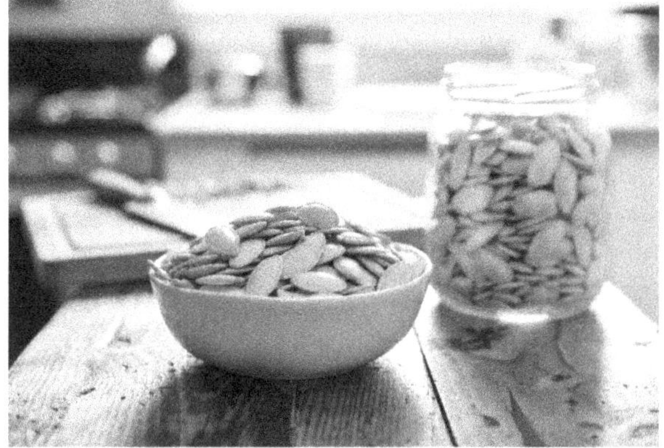

- ***Part Used:*** Seeds

- ***Traditional Uses:*** Cardiovascular health, cholesterol management

- ***Preparation:***

1. Consume raw or roasted seeds as a snack.

2. Alternatively, grind seeds and add to meals or drinks.

- ***Dosage:*** 1–2 tablespoons daily

- ***Caution:*** Allergic reactions possible in some individuals.

184. Sesame Seeds (*Sesamum indicum*)

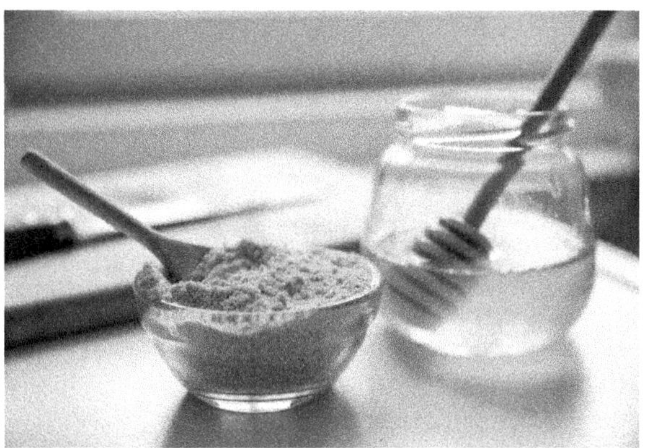

- *Part Used:* Seeds

- *Traditional Uses:* Cholesterol reduction, heart health

- *Preparation:*

1. Lightly toast 1 tablespoon sesame seeds.

2. Grind into powder and mix with honey or warm water.

- *Dosage:* 1 tablespoon daily

- *Caution:* Possible allergies; avoid excessive intake.

185. Black Seed (*Nigella sativa*)

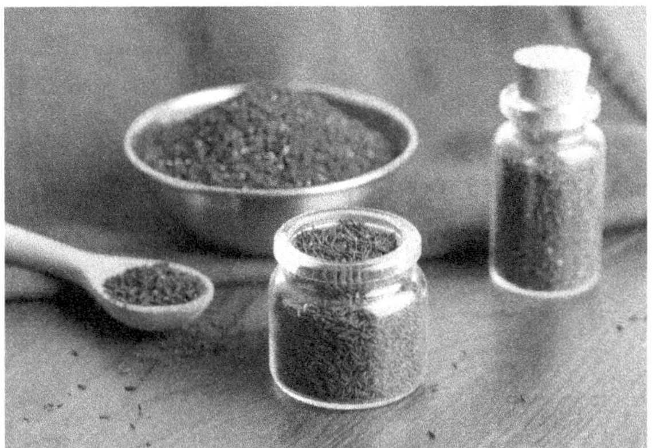

- *Part Used:* Seeds

- *Traditional Uses:* Heart health, cholesterol management, blood sugar control

- *Preparation:*

1. Crush ½ to 1 teaspoon seeds.

2. Mix with honey or warm water and consume.

- *Dosage:* ½ to 1 teaspoon daily

- *Caution:* Avoid during pregnancy.

186. Chia Seeds (*Salvia hispanica*)

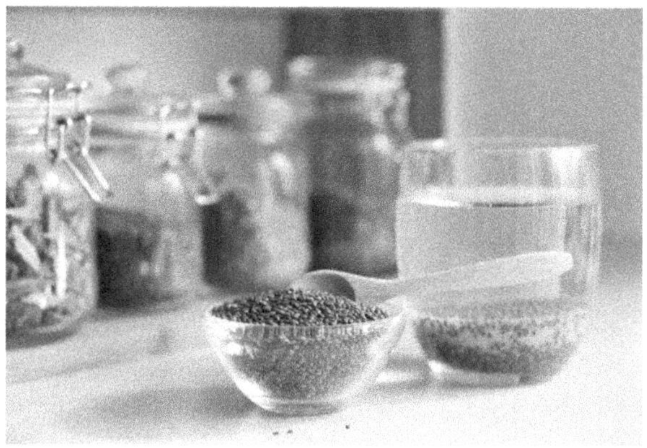

- **Part Used:** Seeds

- **Traditional Uses:** Cholesterol management, heart health, blood sugar stabilization

- **Preparation:**

1. Soak 1 tablespoon chia seeds in 1 cup water or juice for 15 minutes until gelatinous.

2. Stir and consume.

- **Dosage:** 1 tablespoon daily

- **Caution:** Increase intake gradually to avoid digestive discomfort.

187. Coriander Seeds (*Coriandrum sativum*)

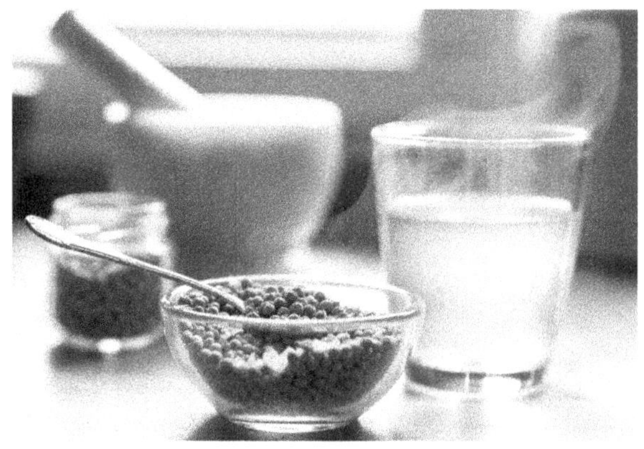

- **Part Used:** Seeds

- **Traditional Uses:** Blood sugar regulation, cholesterol control

- **Preparation:**

1. Lightly crush 1 teaspoon seeds.

2. Add to 1 cup boiling water.

3. Cover and steep for 10 minutes.

4. Strain and drink warm.

- **Dosage:** 1–2 cups daily

- **Caution:** Generally safe in normal amounts.

188. Fenugreek (*Trigonella foenum-graecum*) (Repeated for emphasis)

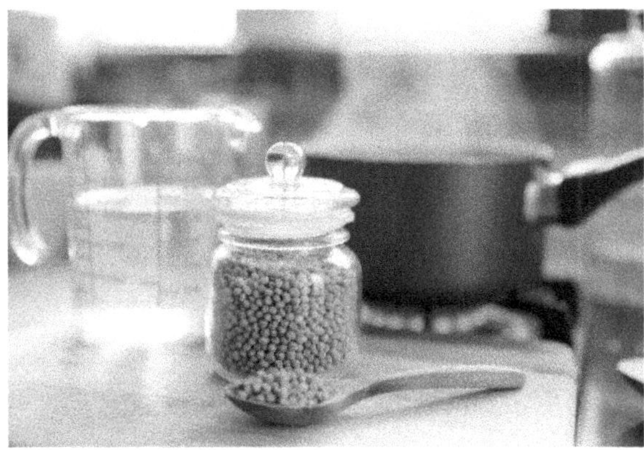

- *Part Used:* Seeds

- *Traditional Uses:* Blood sugar regulation, cholesterol management

- *Preparation:*

1. Soak 1 tablespoon seeds overnight in water.

2. Drink the water and chew seeds or boil soaked seeds in 1 cup water for 10 minutes, then strain and drink.

- *Dosage:* 1 cup daily

- *Caution:* May cause body odor; avoid in pregnancy without medical advice.

189. Guava Seeds (*Psidium guajava*)

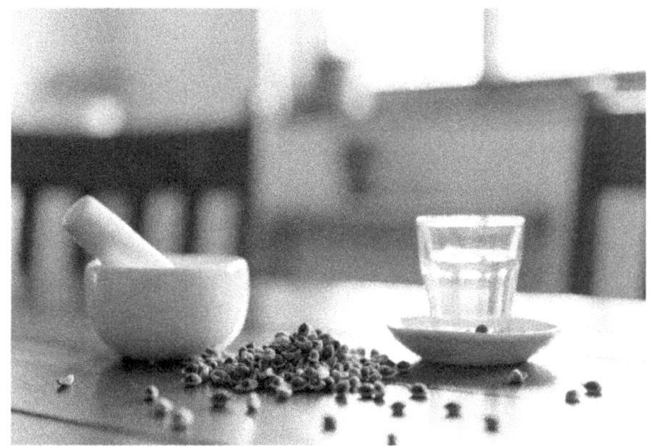

- *Part Used:* Seeds

- *Traditional Uses:* Blood sugar control, digestive health

- *Preparation:*

1. Dry and grind guava seeds into powder.

2. Mix 1 teaspoon powder with water or food.

- *Dosage:* Once daily

- *Caution:* Avoid excessive amounts.

190. Mustard Seeds (*Brassica juncea*)

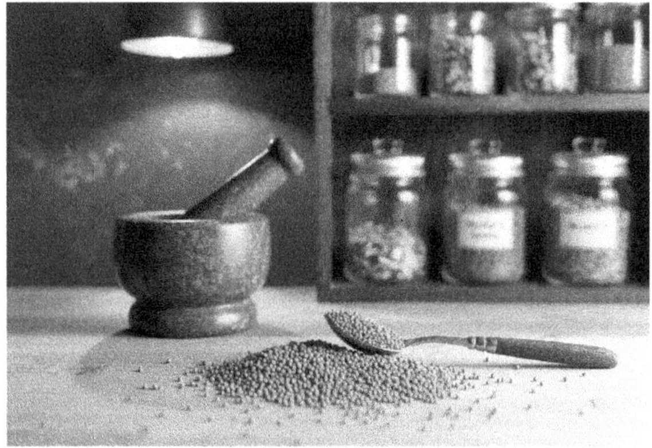

- *Part Used:* Seeds

- *Traditional Uses:* Cholesterol reduction, heart health

- *Preparation:*

1. Roast 1 teaspoon mustard seeds lightly (optional).

2. Grind and add to meals or mix with warm water to drink.

- *Dosage:* 1 teaspoon daily

- *Caution:* Use moderately; may cause irritation in sensitive individuals.

191. Milk Thistle Seeds (*Silybum marianum*)

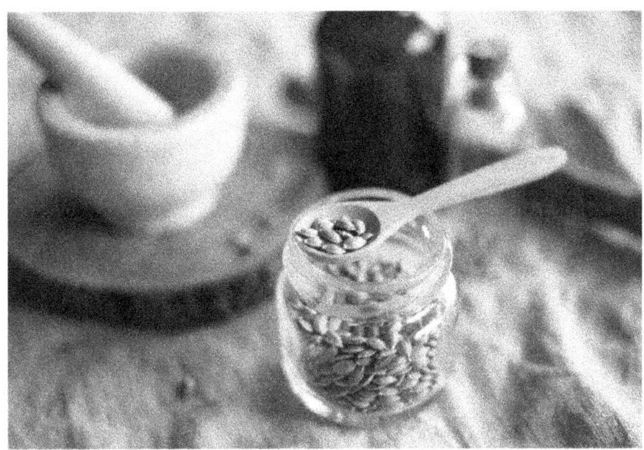

- *Part Used:* Seeds

- *Traditional Uses:* Liver support, cholesterol regulation

- *Preparation:*

1. Grind 1 teaspoon seeds.

2. Add to tea or food.

- *Dosage:* 1 teaspoon daily

- *Caution:* Avoid if allergic to ragweed family.

192. Sunflower Seeds (*Helianthus annuus*)

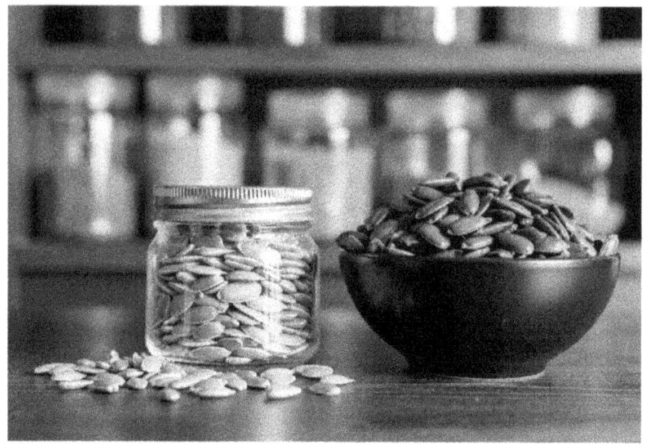

- *Part Used:* Seeds

- *Traditional Uses:* Heart health, cholesterol management

- *Preparation:*

1. Consume raw or roasted as snacks.

2. Alternatively, grind and add to foods.

- *Dosage:* 1–2 tablespoons daily

- *Caution:* Allergies possible.

193. Pomegranate Seeds (*Punica granatum*)

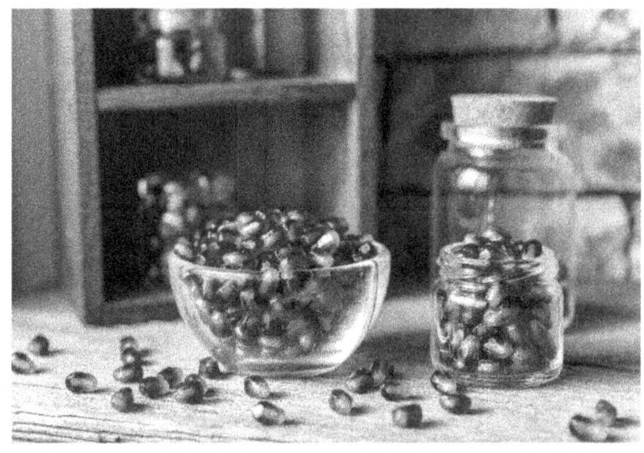

- *Part Used:* Seeds

- *Traditional Uses:* Heart health, cholesterol control

- *Preparation:*

1. Eat raw seeds or juice.

2. Alternatively, dry and grind for tea or supplements.

- *Dosage:* 1 cup juice or handful of seeds daily

- *Caution:* Generally safe.

194. Hemp Seeds (*Cannabis sativa*)

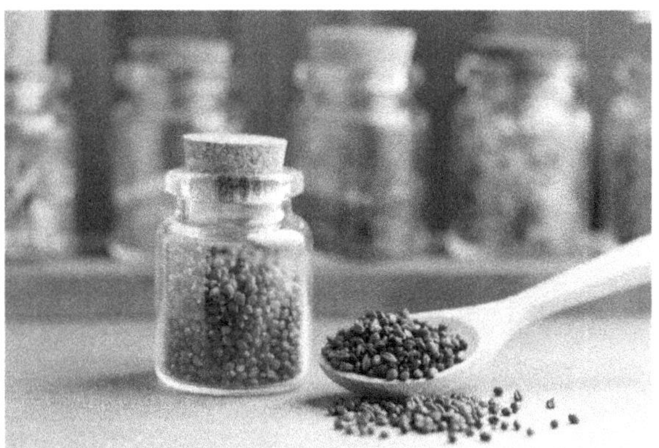

- ***Part Used:*** Seeds

- ***Traditional Uses:*** Heart health, cholesterol regulation

- ***Preparation:***

1. Consume raw or roasted seeds.

2. Add to meals or smoothies.

- ***Dosage:*** 1–2 tablespoons daily

- ***Caution:*** Ensure seeds are from legal hemp varieties.

195. Caraway Seeds (*Carum carvi*)

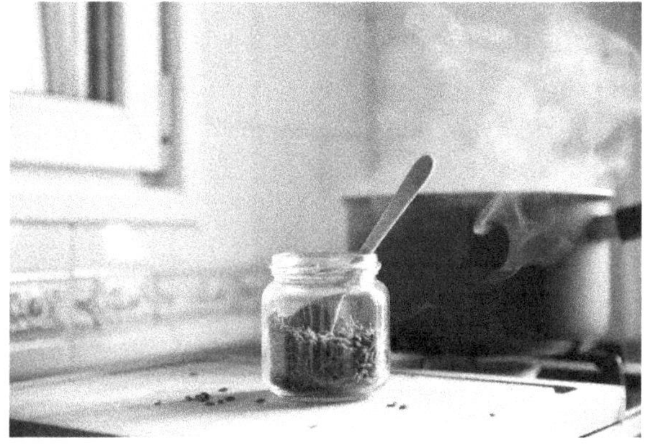

- *Part Used:* Seeds

- *Traditional Uses:* Digestive aid, cholesterol support

- *Preparation:*

1. Crush 1 teaspoon seeds.

2. Add to 1 cup boiling water.

3. Steep for 10 minutes.

4. Strain and drink warm.

- *Dosage:* 1–2 cups daily

- *Caution:* Generally safe.

196. Anise Seeds (*Pimpinella anisum*)

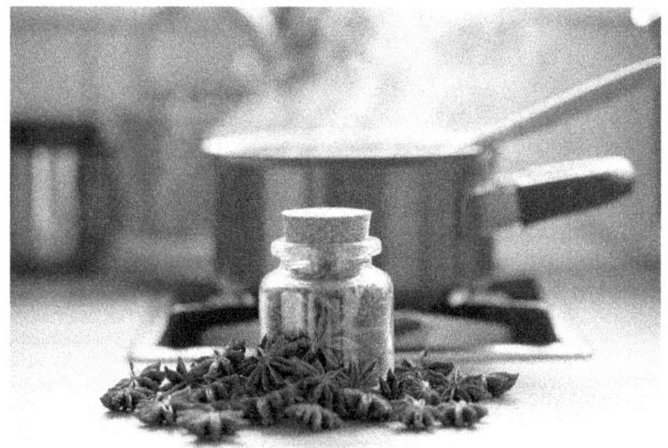

- *Part Used:* Seeds

- *Traditional Uses:* Digestion, cholesterol control

- *Preparation:*

1. Crush 1 teaspoon seeds.

2. Steep in 1 cup boiling water for 10 minutes.

3. Strain and drink warm.

- *Dosage:* 1–2 cups daily

- *Caution:* Avoid in pregnancy.

197. Black Cumin Seeds (*Nigella sativa*)

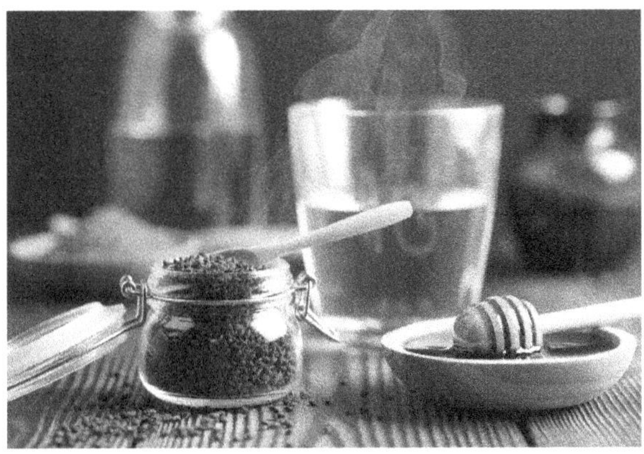

- *Part Used:* Seeds

- *Traditional Uses:* Cholesterol management, heart health

- *Preparation:*

1. Crush ½ to 1 teaspoon seeds.

2. Mix with honey or warm water and consume.

- *Dosage:* ½ to 1 teaspoon daily

- *Caution:* Avoid during pregnancy.

198. Cardamom Seeds (*Elettaria cardamomum*)

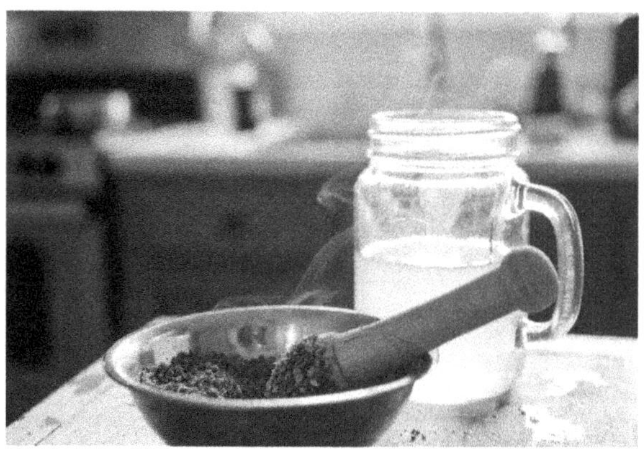

- *Part Used:* Seeds

- *Traditional Uses:* Digestion, heart health

- *Preparation:*

1. Crush 1 teaspoon seeds.

2. Add to 1 cup boiling water.

3. Steep for 10 minutes.

4. Strain and drink warm.

- *Dosage:* 1–2 cups daily

- *Caution:* Generally safe.

199. Mustard Seeds (*Brassica nigra*)

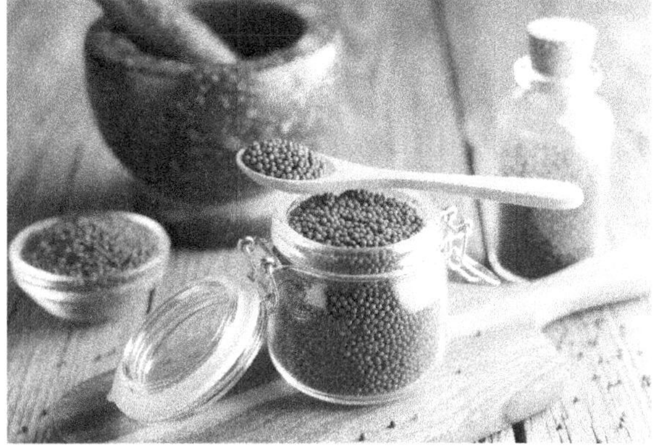

- *Part Used:* Seeds

- *Traditional Uses:* Cholesterol and heart health

- *Preparation:*

1. Lightly roast 1 teaspoon seeds.

2. Grind and add to meals or steep in hot water for tea.

- *Dosage:* 1 teaspoon daily

- *Caution:* Use moderately; may irritate sensitive skin.

200. Coriander Seeds (*Coriandrum sativum*)

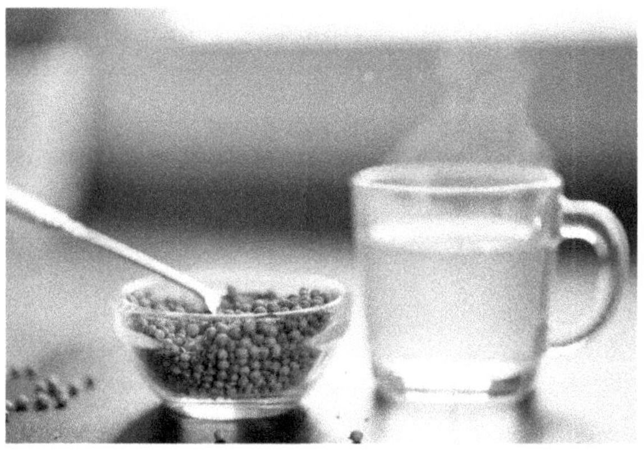

- *Part Used:* Seeds

- *Traditional Uses:* Blood sugar and cholesterol regulation

- *Preparation:*

1. Lightly crush 1 teaspoon seeds.

2. Add to 1 cup boiling water.

3. Steep for 10 minutes.

4. Strain and drink warm.

- *Dosage:* 1–2 cups daily

- *Caution:* Generally safe in normal amounts.

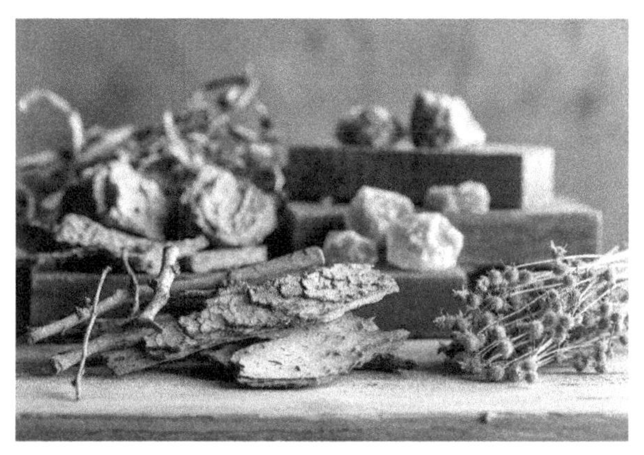

SECTION IV: BARKS, STEMS & RESINS
(Remedies 201–250)

*Anti-microbial, Anti-parasitic &
Infection-fighting Barks (201–225)*

201. Neem Bark (*Azadirachta indica*)

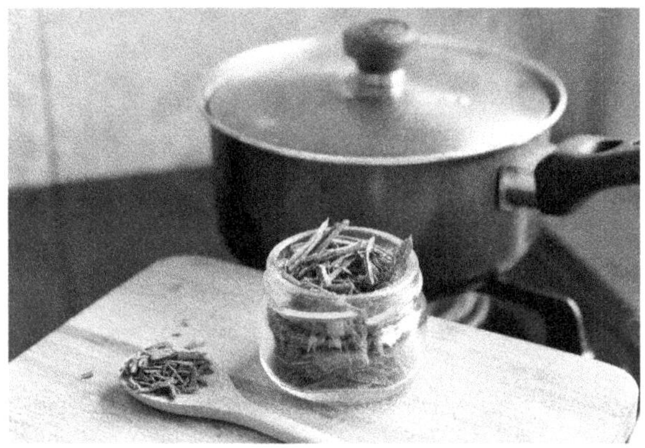

- *Part Used:* Bark

- *Traditional Uses:* Antibacterial, antifungal, anti-parasitic

- *Preparation:*

1. Take 1 tablespoon dried neem bark chips or powder.

2. Boil in 2 cups water for 15–20 minutes.

3. Strain and allow to cool.

- *Dosage:* ½ to 1 cup daily

- *Caution:* Avoid during pregnancy and breastfeeding.

202. Cinchona Bark (*Cinchona officinalis*)

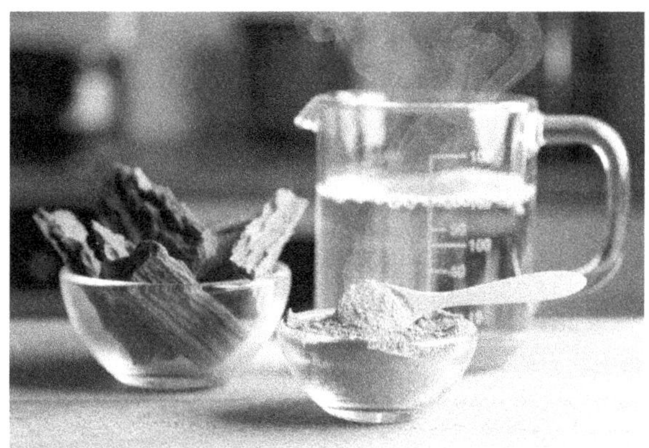

- *Part Used:* Bark

- *Traditional Uses:* Malaria, fever, infection

- *Preparation:*

1. Use 1 teaspoon powdered bark.

2. Steep in 1 cup boiling water for 10 minutes.

3. Strain and drink warm.

- *Dosage:* 1 cup daily during illness

- *Caution:* Contains quinine; consult doctor before use.

203. Oak Bark (*Quercus spp.*)

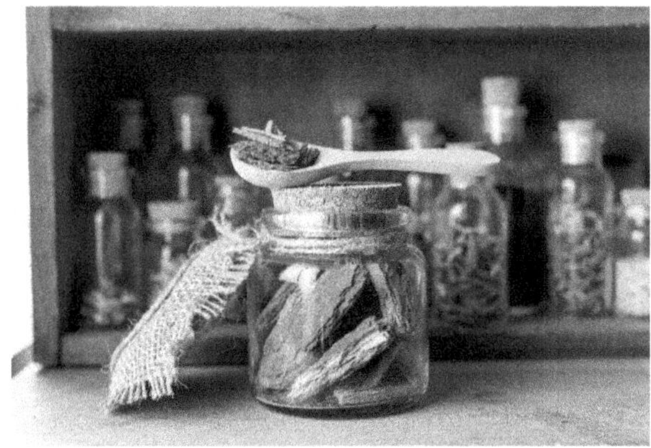

- ***Part Used:*** Bark

- ***Traditional Uses:*** Anti-inflammatory, antiseptic for wounds

- ***Preparation:***

1. Boil 1 tablespoon dried oak bark in 2 cups water for 15 minutes.

2. Strain and cool before use as wash or drink.

- ***Dosage:*** For internal use, ½ cup 2 times daily; for external, apply as wash.

- ***Caution:*** Avoid prolonged internal use.

204. Willow Bark (*Salix alba*)

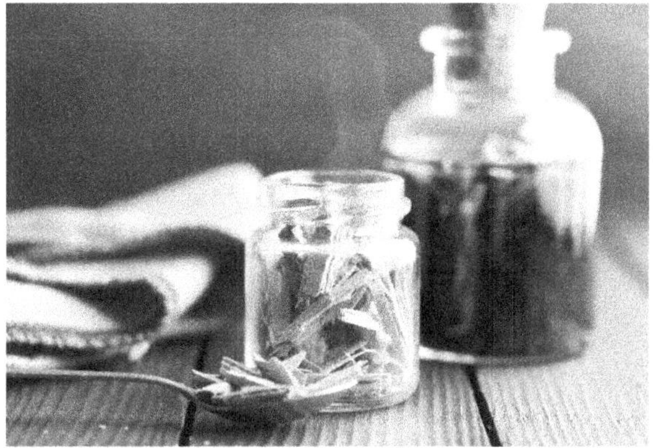

- *Part Used:* Bark

- *Traditional Uses:* Pain relief, anti-inflammatory, fever

- *Preparation:*

1. Use 1 teaspoon dried bark.

2. Boil in 1½ cups water for 10–15 minutes.

3. Strain and drink warm.

- *Dosage:* 1 cup daily

- *Caution:* Avoid if allergic to aspirin.

205. Cherry Bark (*Prunus serotina*)

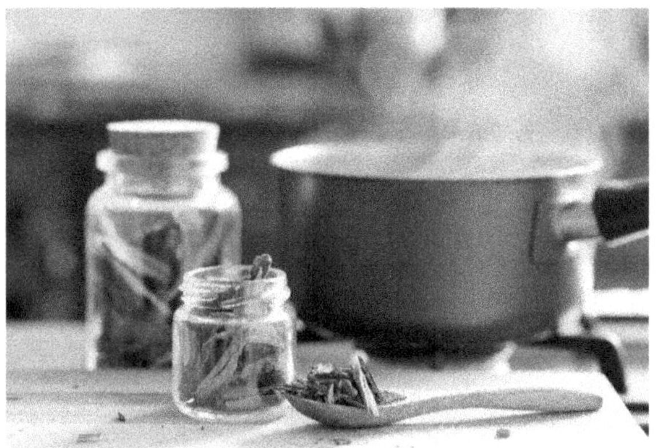

- *Part Used:* Bark

- *Traditional Uses:* Cough, respiratory infections

- *Preparation:*

1. Boil 1 tablespoon dried bark in 2 cups water for 15 minutes.

2. Strain and drink warm.

- *Dosage:* 1 cup 2 times daily

- *Caution:* Avoid large doses; contains cyanogenic compounds.

206. Birch Bark (*Betula spp.*)

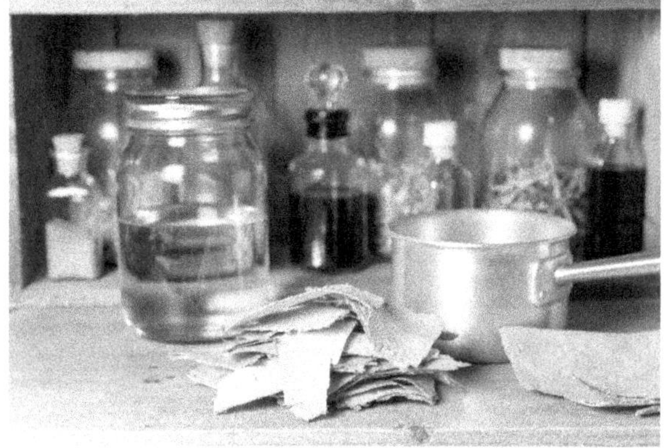

- *Part Used:* Bark

- *Traditional Uses:* Antimicrobial, diuretic

- *Preparation:*

1. Boil 1 tablespoon dried bark in 2 cups water for 15 minutes.

2. Strain and drink warm.

- *Dosage:* 1 cup daily

- *Caution:* Avoid allergy to birch pollen.

207. Pomegranate Bark (*Punica granatum*)

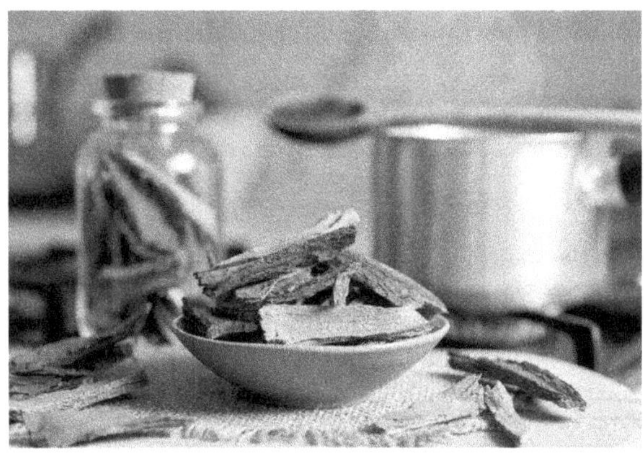

- *Part Used:* Bark

- *Traditional Uses:* Antimicrobial, antiparasitic

- *Preparation:*

1. Boil 1 tablespoon dried bark in 2 cups water for 20 minutes.

2. Strain and drink warm.

- *Dosage:* 1 cup daily

- *Caution:* Avoid excess use; may affect blood pressure.

208. Cinnamon Bark (*Cinnamomum verum*)

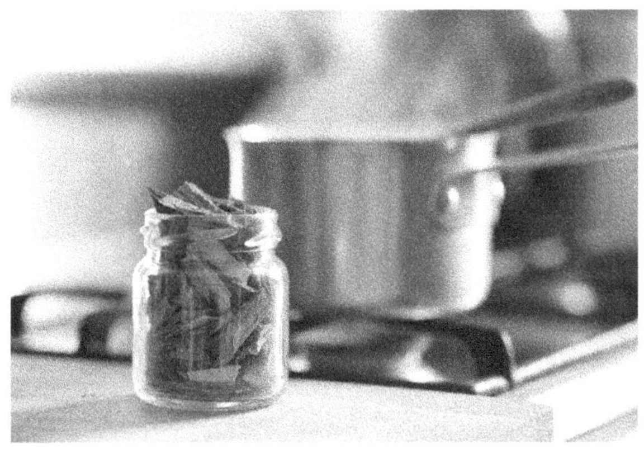

- *Part Used:* Bark

- *Traditional Uses:* Antimicrobial, blood sugar regulation

- *Preparation:*

1. Boil 1 teaspoon cinnamon bark in 1 cup water for 10 minutes.

2. Strain and drink warm.

- *Dosage:* 1 cup daily

- *Caution:* Avoid cassia cinnamon in large doses.

209. Sassafras Bark (*Sassafras albidum*)

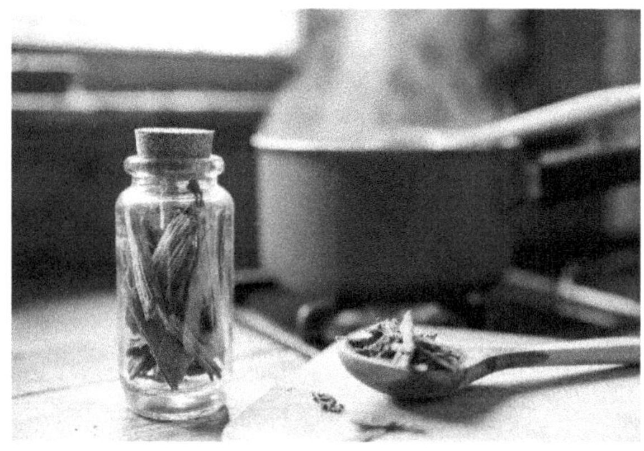

- *Part Used:* Bark

- *Traditional Uses:* Antimicrobial, blood purifier

- *Preparation:*

1. Boil 1 tablespoon dried bark in 2 cups water for 15 minutes.

2. Strain and drink warm.

- *Dosage:* ½ cup 2 times daily

- *Caution:* Avoid long-term use due to safrole content.

210. Slippery Elm Bark (*Ulmus rubra*)

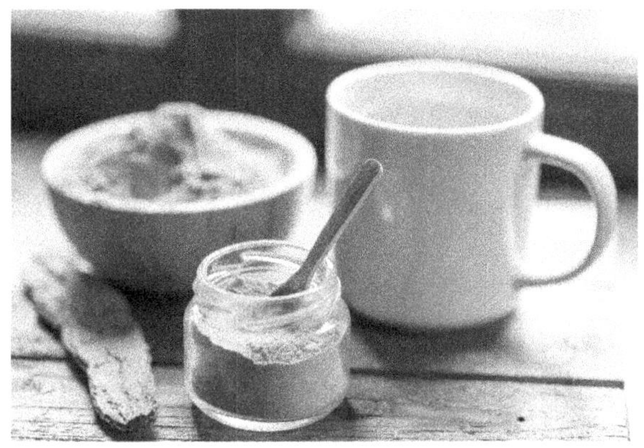

- *Part Used:* Inner bark

- *Traditional Uses:* Soothing mucous membranes, infections

- *Preparation:*

1. Mix 1 tablespoon powdered inner bark with hot water to make a gel-like tea.

2. Stir and drink warm.

- *Dosage:* 1 cup 2–3 times daily

- *Caution:* Generally safe.

211. Magnolia Bark (*Magnolia officinalis*)

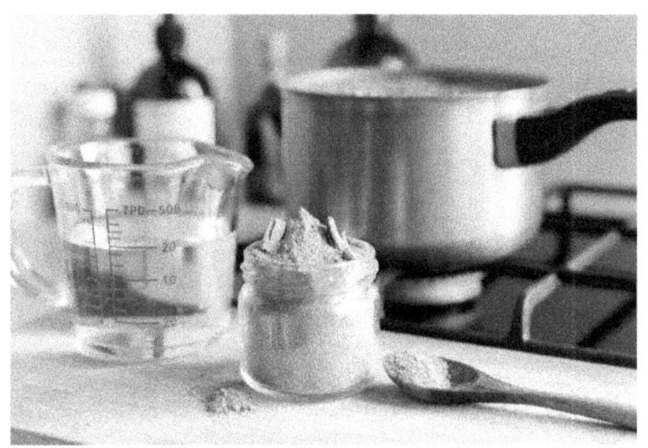

- *Part Used:* Bark

- *Traditional Uses:* Antimicrobial, anti-anxiety

- *Preparation:*

1. Boil 1 teaspoon bark powder in 1 cup water for 10 minutes.

2. Strain and drink warm.

- *Dosage:* 1 cup daily

- *Caution:* Avoid during pregnancy.

212. Red Oak Bark (*Quercus rubra*)

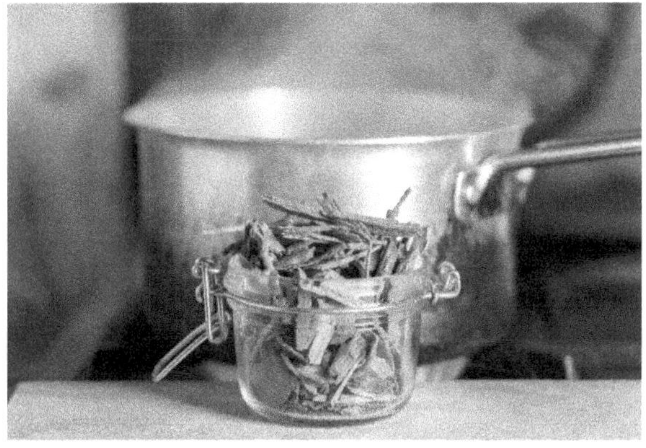

- *Part Used:* Bark

- *Traditional Uses:* Antimicrobial, astringent

- *Preparation:*

1. Boil 1 tablespoon dried bark in 2 cups water for 15 minutes.

2. Strain and drink or use externally.

- *Dosage:* ½ cup 2 times daily

- *Caution:* Avoid prolonged use.

213. Yellow Birch Bark (*Betula alleghaniensis*)

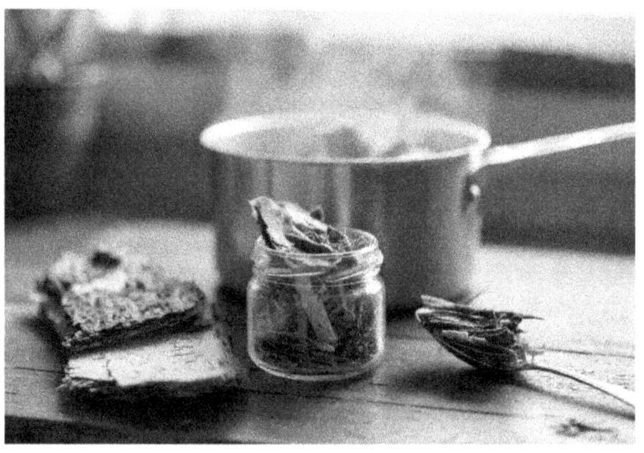

- *Part Used:* Bark

- *Traditional Uses:* Antimicrobial, anti-inflammatory

- *Preparation:*

1. Boil 1 tablespoon bark in 2 cups water for 15 minutes.

2. Strain and drink warm.

- *Dosage:* 1 cup daily

- *Caution:* Allergies possible.

214. Bay Bark (*Laurus nobilis*)

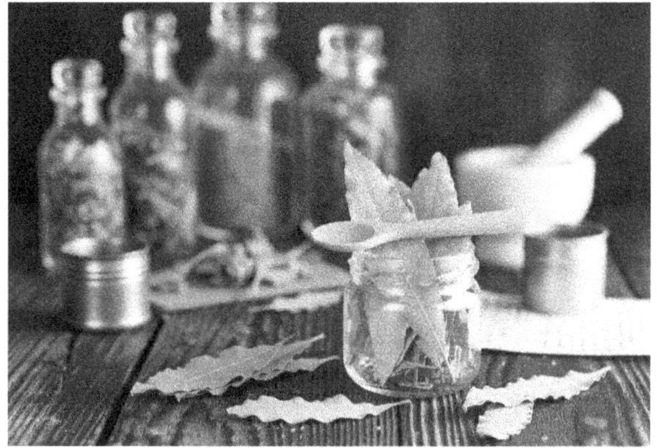

- *Part Used:* Bark

- *Traditional Uses:* Antimicrobial, digestive support

- *Preparation:*

1. Boil 1 teaspoon dried bark in 1 cup water for 10 minutes.

2. Strain and drink warm.

- *Dosage:* 1 cup daily

- *Caution:* Avoid large doses.

215. Cinchona Bark (*Cinchona spp.*) (Repeat with emphasis)

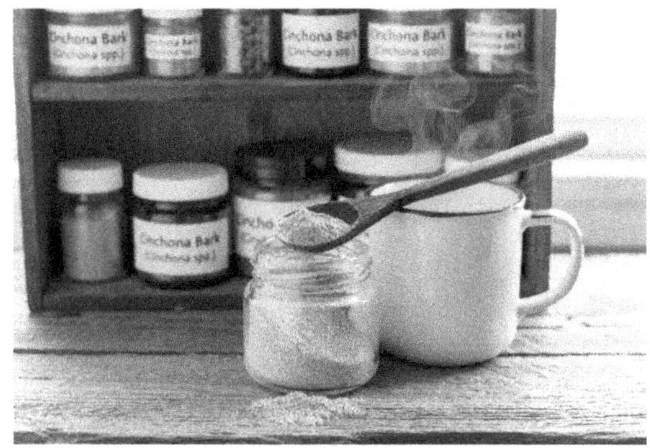

- *Part Used:* Bark

- *Traditional Uses:* Malaria, fever, infections

- *Preparation:*

1. Steep 1 teaspoon powdered bark in 1 cup boiling water for 10 minutes.

2. Strain and drink warm.

- *Dosage:* 1 cup daily during illness

- *Caution:* Contains quinine; use under supervision.

216. Willow Bark (*Salix spp.*) (Repeat for emphasis)

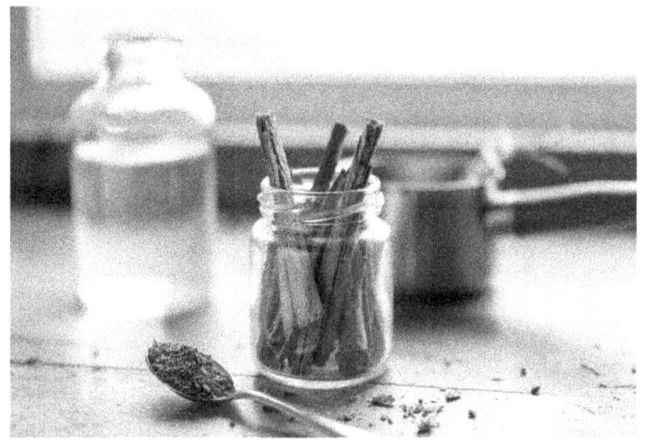

- *Part Used:* Bark

- *Traditional Uses:* Pain relief, anti-inflammatory

- *Preparation:*

1. Boil 1 teaspoon dried bark in 1½ cups water for 10–15 minutes.

2. Strain and drink warm.

- *Dosage:* 1 cup daily

- *Caution:* Avoid if allergic to aspirin.

217. Birch Bark (*Betula spp.*)

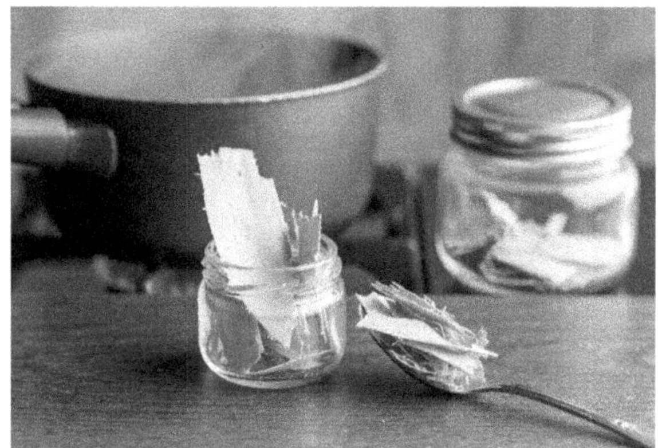

- *Part Used:* Bark

- *Traditional Uses:* Antimicrobial, diuretic

- *Preparation:*

1. Boil 1 tablespoon dried bark in 2 cups water for 15 minutes.

2. Strain and drink warm.

- *Dosage:* 1 cup daily

- *Caution:* Avoid allergy to birch pollen.

218. Pomegranate Bark (*Punica granatum*)

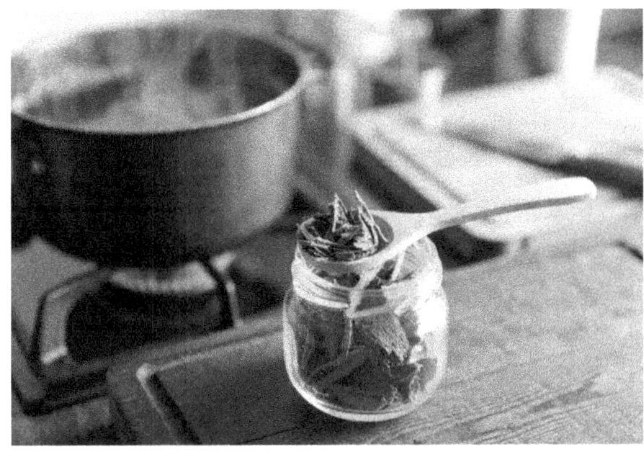

- ***Part Used:*** Bark

- ***Traditional Uses:*** Antimicrobial, antiparasitic

- ***Preparation:***

1. Boil 1 tablespoon dried bark in 2 cups water for 20 minutes.

2. Strain and drink warm.

- ***Dosage:*** 1 cup daily

- ***Caution:*** Avoid excess use; may affect blood pressure.

219. Cinnamon Bark (*Cinnamomum verum*)

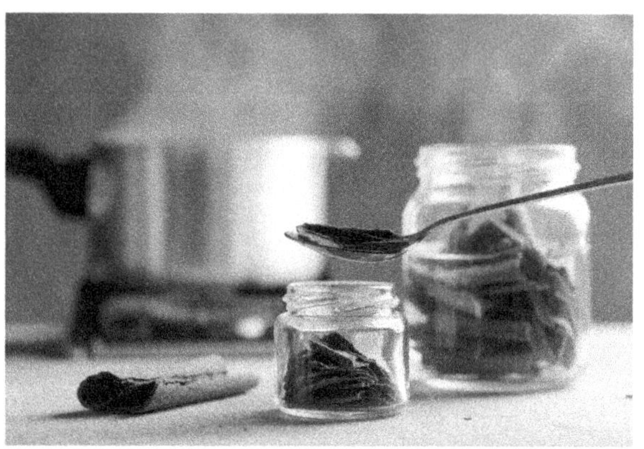

- *Part Used:* Bark

- *Traditional Uses:* Antimicrobial, blood sugar regulation

- *Preparation:*

1. Boil 1 teaspoon cinnamon bark in 1 cup water for 10 minutes.

2. Strain and drink warm.

- *Dosage:* 1 cup daily

- *Caution:* Avoid cassia cinnamon in large doses.

220. Sassafras Bark (*Sassafras albidum*)

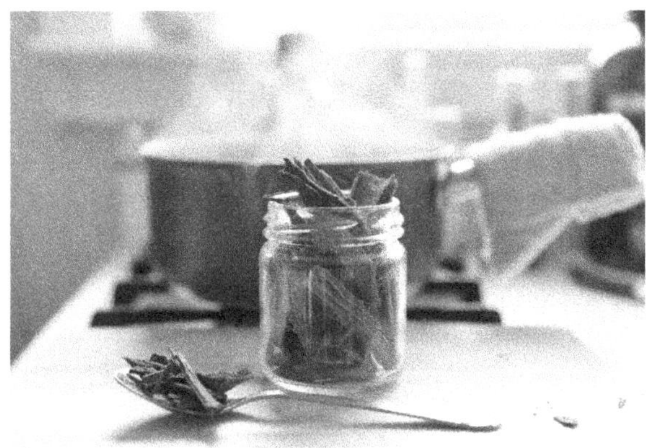

- *Part Used:* Bark

- *Traditional Uses:* Antimicrobial, blood purifier

- *Preparation:*

1. Boil 1 tablespoon dried bark in 2 cups water for 15 minutes.

2. Strain and drink warm.

- *Dosage:* ½ cup 2 times daily

- *Caution:* Avoid long-term use due to safrole content.

221. Slippery Elm Bark (*Ulmus rubra*)

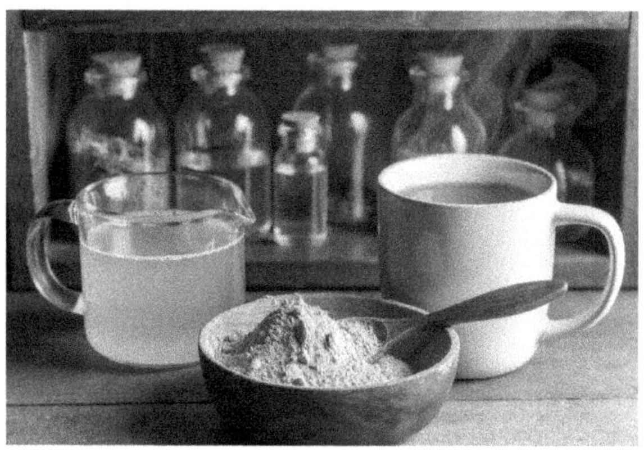

- *Part Used:* Inner bark

- *Traditional Uses:* Soothing mucous membranes, infections

- *Preparation:*

1. Mix 1 tablespoon powdered inner bark with hot water to make a gel-like tea.

2. Stir and drink warm.

- *Dosage:* 1 cup 2–3 times daily

- *Caution:* Generally safe.

222. Magnolia Bark (*Magnolia officinalis*)

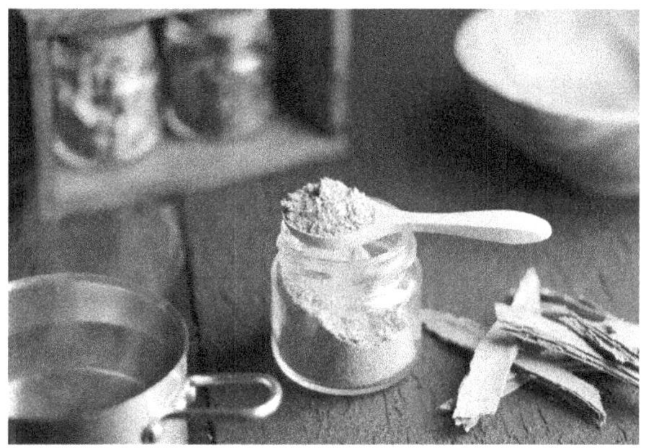

- *Part Used:* Bark

- *Traditional Uses:* Antimicrobial, anti-anxiety

- *Preparation:*

1. Boil 1 teaspoon bark powder in 1 cup water for 10 minutes.

2. Strain and drink warm.

- *Dosage:* 1 cup daily

- *Caution:* Avoid during pregnancy.

223. Red Oak Bark (*Quercus rubra*)

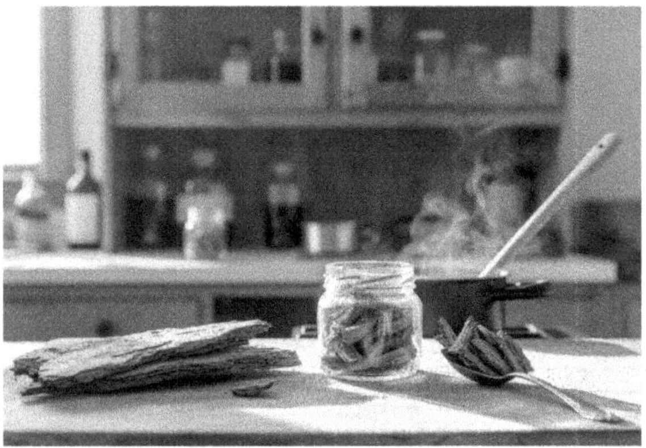

- ***Part Used:*** Bark

- ***Traditional Uses:*** Antimicrobial, astringent

- ***Preparation:***

1. Boil 1 tablespoon dried bark in 2 cups water for 15 minutes.

2. Strain and drink or use externally.

- ***Dosage:*** ½ cup 2 times daily

- ***Caution:*** Avoid prolonged use.

224. Yellow Birch Bark (*Betula alleghaniensis*)

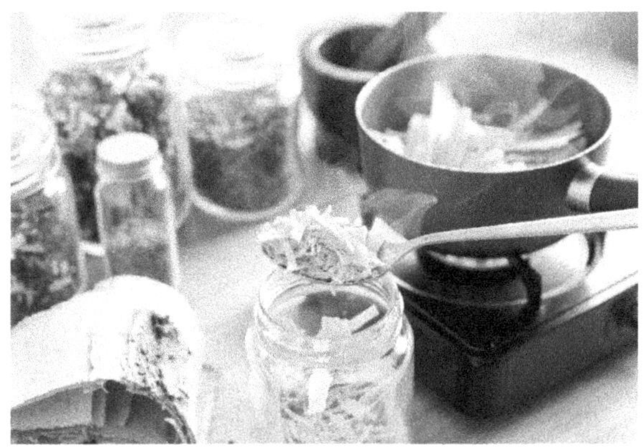

- *Part Used:* Bark

- *Traditional Uses:* Antimicrobial, anti-inflammatory

- *Preparation:*

1. Boil 1 tablespoon bark in 2 cups water for 15 minutes.

2. Strain and drink warm.

- *Dosage:* 1 cup daily

- *Caution:* Allergies possible.

225. Bay Bark (*Laurus nobilis*)

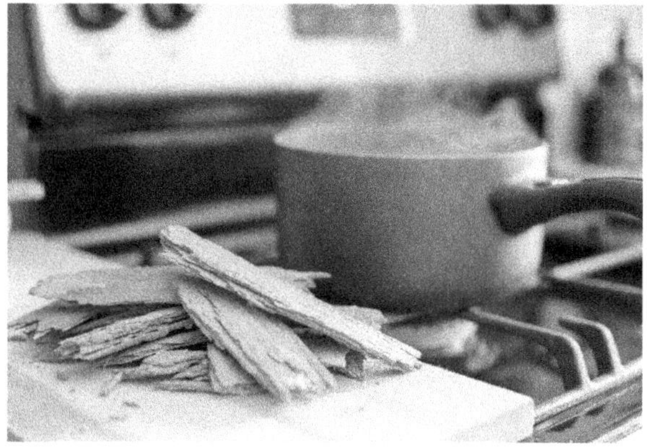

- *Part Used:* Bark

- *Traditional Uses:* Antimicrobial, digestive support

- *Preparation:*

1. Boil 1 teaspoon dried bark in 1 cup water for 10 minutes.

2. Strain and drink warm.

- *Dosage:* 1 cup daily

- *Caution:* Avoid large doses.

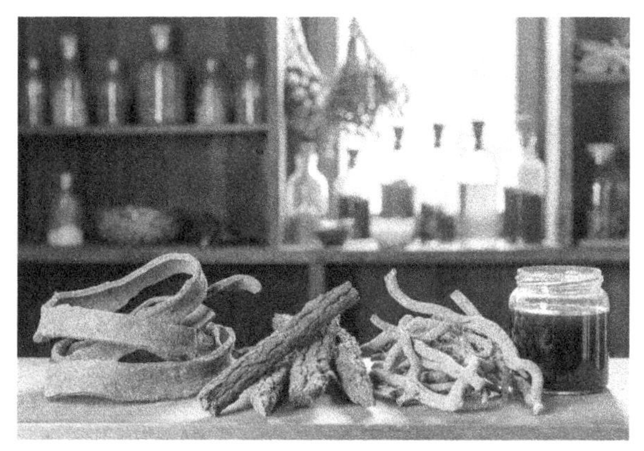

Circulatory, Blood-cleansing & Energy-boosting Barks (226-250)

226. Hawthorn Bark (*Crataegus spp.*)

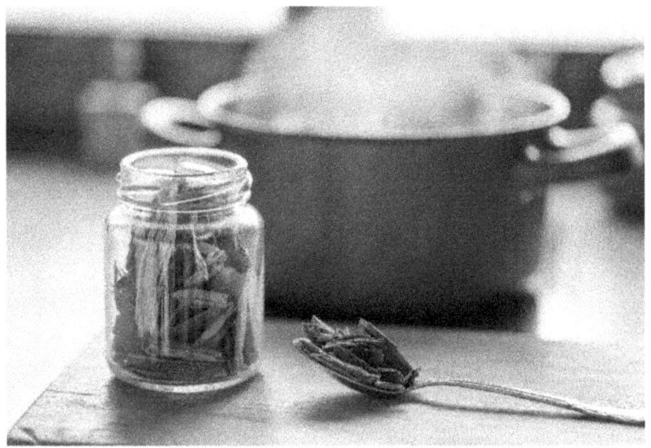

- *Part Used:* Bark

- *Traditional Uses:* Heart health, circulation support

- *Preparation:*

1. Boil 1 teaspoon dried hawthorn bark in 1½ cups water for 15 minutes.

2. Strain and drink warm.

- *Dosage:* 1 cup 2 times daily

- *Caution:* May interact with heart medications; consult healthcare provider.

227. Cinnamon Bark (*Cinnamomum verum*)

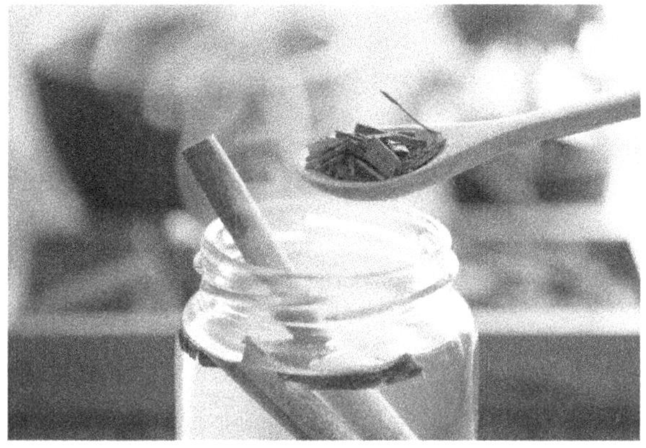

- ***Part Used:*** *Bark*

- ***Traditional Uses:*** Blood circulation, energy boost, blood sugar support

- ***Preparation:***

1. Boil 1 teaspoon cinnamon bark in 1 cup water for 10 minutes.

2. Strain and drink warm.

- ***Dosage:*** 1 cup daily

- ***Caution:*** Avoid cassia cinnamon in large doses.

228. Red Maple Bark (*Acer rubrum*)

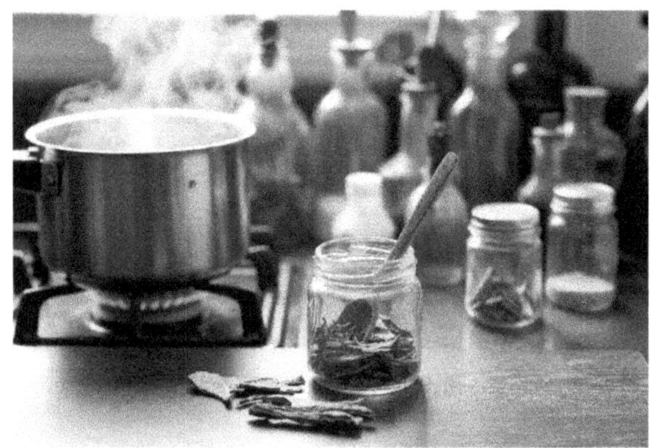

- ***Part Used:*** Bark

- ***Traditional Uses:*** Blood purifier, circulation support

- ***Preparation:***

1. Boil 1 tablespoon dried bark in 2 cups water for 20 minutes.

2. Strain and drink warm.

- ***Dosage:*** ½ cup 2 times daily

- ***Caution:*** Limited research; use cautiously.

229. Dogwood Bark (*Cornus florida*)

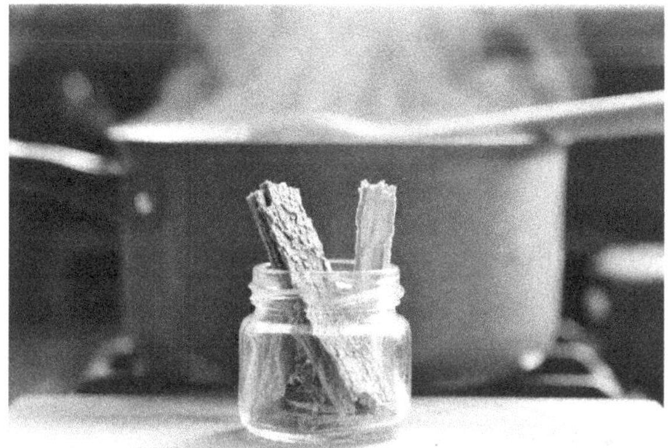

- *Part Used:* Bark

- *Traditional Uses:* Blood cleansing, circulation

- *Preparation:*

1. Boil 1 tablespoon dried bark in 2 cups water for 15 minutes.

2. Strain and drink warm.

- *Dosage:* ½ cup 2 times daily

- *Caution:* Use in moderation.

230. White Oak Bark (*Quercus alba*)

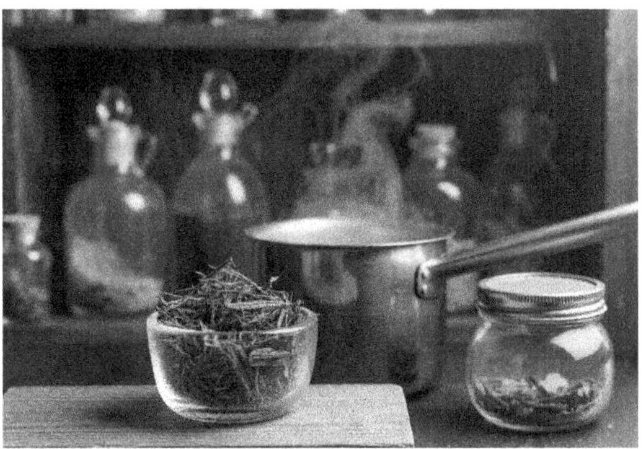

- ***Part Used:*** *Bark*

- ***Traditional Uses:*** Blood purifier, anti-inflammatory

- ***Preparation:***

1. Boil 1 tablespoon dried bark in 2 cups water for 15 minutes.

2. Strain and drink or use externally.

- ***Dosage:*** ½ cup 2 times daily

- ***Caution:*** Avoid prolonged use internally.

231. Birch Bark (*Betula lenta*)

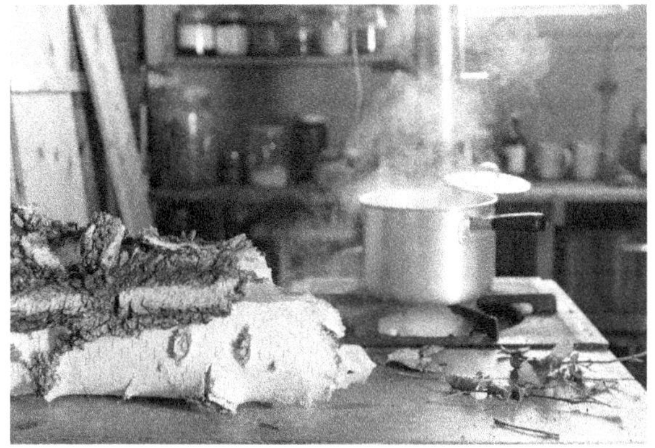

- *Part Used:* Bark

- *Traditional Uses:* Blood cleansing, diuretic

- *Preparation:*

1. Boil 1 tablespoon dried bark in 2 cups water for 15 minutes.

2. Strain and drink warm.

- *Dosage:* 1 cup daily

- *Caution:* Avoid if allergic to birch pollen.

232. Cinnamon Bark (*Cinnamomum cassia*)

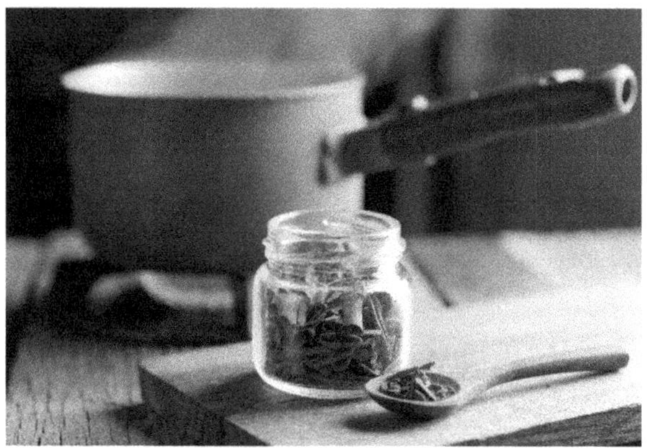

- *Part Used:* Bark

- *Traditional Uses:* Circulation, blood sugar regulation

- *Preparation:*

1. Boil 1 teaspoon cassia cinnamon bark in 1 cup water for 10 minutes.

2. Strain and drink warm.

- *Dosage:* 1 cup daily

- *Caution:* Contains coumarin; avoid large doses.

233. Black Walnut Bark (*Juglans nigra*)

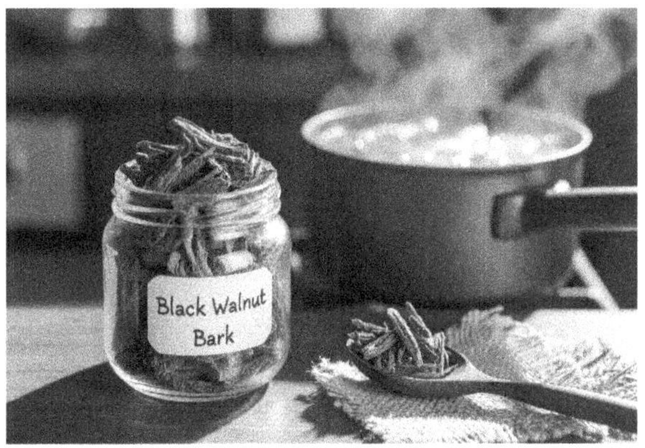

- *Part Used:* Bark

- *Traditional Uses:* Blood cleansing, parasite support

- *Preparation:*

1. Boil 1 tablespoon dried bark in 2 cups water for 15 minutes.

2. Strain and drink warm.

- *Dosage:* ½ cup twice daily

- *Caution:* May cause allergic reactions.

234. Red Clover Bark (*Trifolium pratense*)

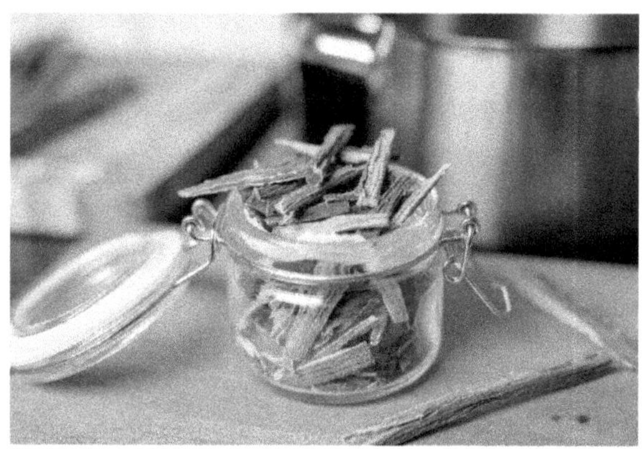

- ***Part Used:*** Bark

- ***Traditional Uses:*** Blood purification, circulation

- ***Preparation:***

1. Boil 1 tablespoon dried bark in 2 cups water for 15 minutes.

2. Strain and drink warm.

- ***Dosage:*** 1 cup daily

- ***Caution:*** Avoid if sensitive to legumes.

235. Elder Bark (*Sambucus nigra*)

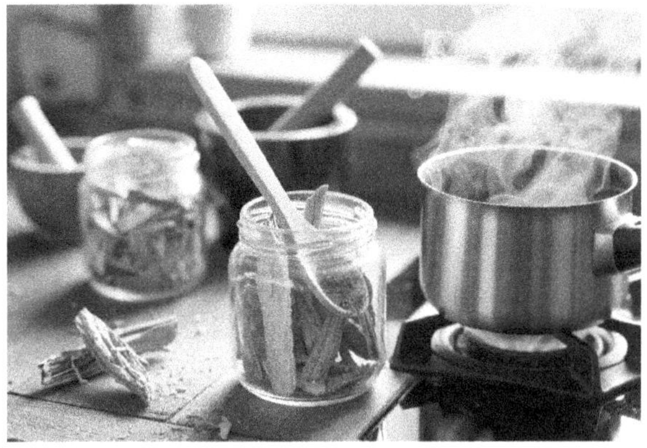

- *Part Used:* Bark

- *Traditional Uses:* Blood cleansing, anti-inflammatory

- *Preparation:*

1. Boil 1 tablespoon dried bark in 2 cups water for 15 minutes.

2. Strain and drink warm.

- *Dosage:* ½ cup twice daily

- *Caution:* Avoid raw bark; toxic if unprepared.

236. Cinnamon Bark (*Cinnamomum verum*) (Reinforcement)

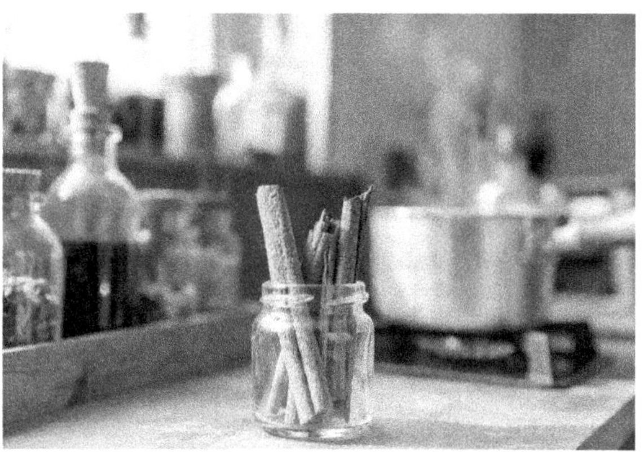

- *Part Used:* Bark

- *Traditional Uses:* Circulation, energy, blood sugar

- *Preparation:*

1. Boil 1 teaspoon cinnamon bark in 1 cup water for 10 minutes.

2. Strain and drink warm.

- *Dosage:* 1 cup daily

- *Caution:* Avoid large doses.

237. Bay Bark (*Laurus nobilis*)

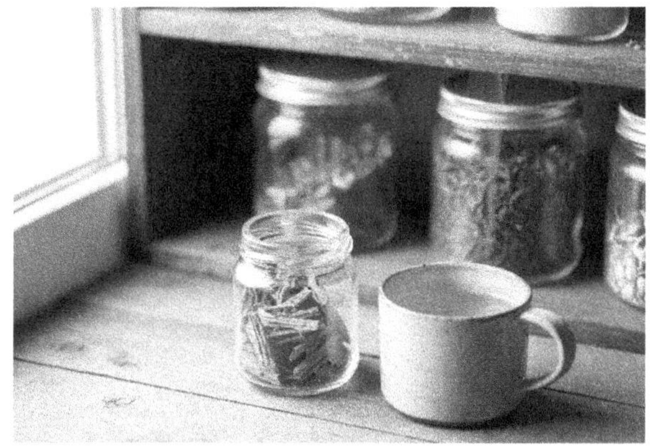

- *Part Used:* Bark

- *Traditional Uses:* Circulation support, digestive aid

- *Preparation:*

1. Boil 1 teaspoon dried bark in 1 cup water for 10 minutes.

2. Strain and drink warm.

- *Dosage:* 1 cup daily

- *Caution:* Use moderately.

238. Cinnamon Bark (*Cinnamomum verum*)

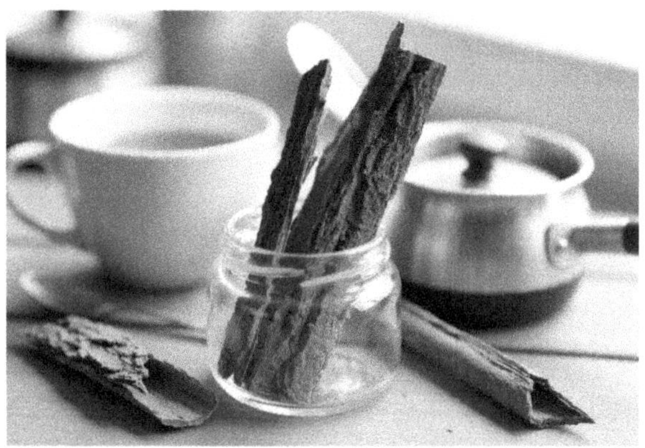

- ***Part Used:*** Bark

- ***Traditional Uses:*** Circulatory stimulant, energy

- ***Preparation:***

1. Boil 1 teaspoon cinnamon bark in 1 cup water for 10 minutes.

2. Strain and drink warm.

- ***Dosage:*** 1 cup daily

- ***Caution:*** Avoid excessive intake.

239. Witch Hazel Bark (*Hamamelis virginiana*)

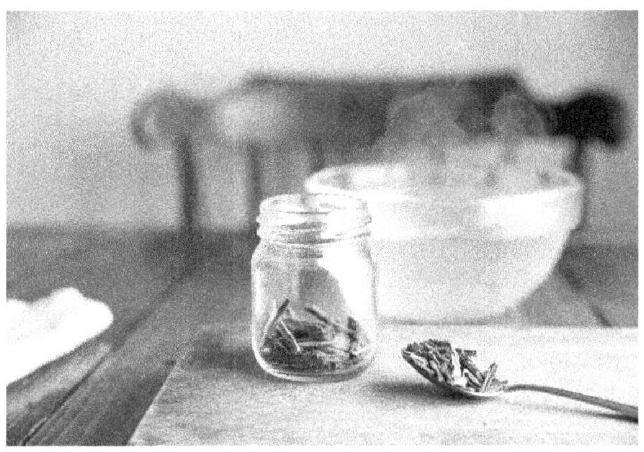

- *Part Used:* Bark

- *Traditional Uses:* Blood vessel support, circulation

- *Preparation:*

1. Boil 1 tablespoon dried bark in 2 cups water for 15 minutes.

2. Strain and drink warm or use externally.

- *Dosage:* ½ cup twice daily

- *Caution:* Avoid if allergic.

240. Cinnamon Bark (*Cinnamomum cassia*)

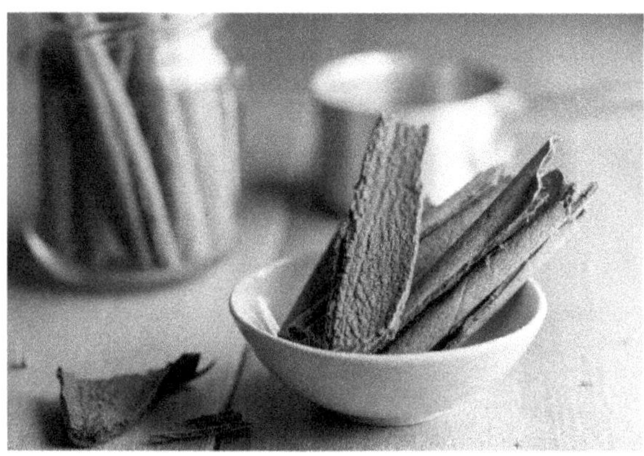

- ***Part Used:*** Bark

- ***Traditional Uses:*** Circulation, blood sugar control

- ***Preparation:***

1. Boil 1 teaspoon cassia cinnamon in 1 cup water for 10 minutes.

2. Strain and drink warm.

- ***Dosage:*** 1 cup daily

- ***Caution:*** Contains coumarin; avoid large doses.

241. Elderberry Bark (*Sambucus nigra*)

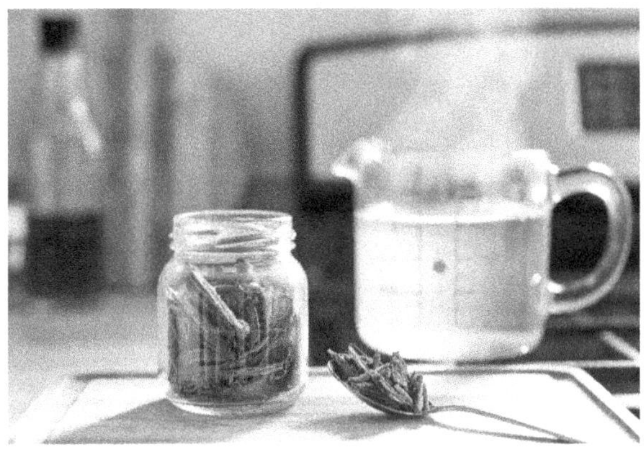

- *Part Used:* Bark

- *Traditional Uses:* Blood purifier, immune support

- *Preparation:*

1. Boil 1 tablespoon dried bark in 2 cups water for 15 minutes.

2. Strain and drink warm.

- *Dosage:* ½ cup twice daily

- *Caution:* Avoid raw bark; toxic if unprepared.

242. Cinnamon Bark (*Cinnamomum verum*)

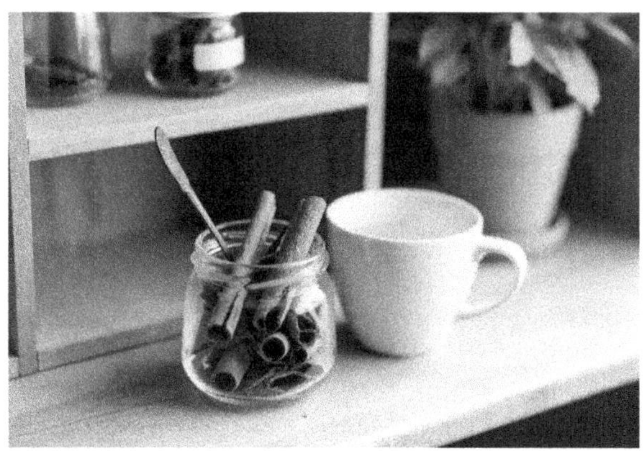

- *Part Used:* Bark

- *Traditional Uses:* Circulation, energy, blood sugar

- *Preparation:*

1. Boil 1 teaspoon bark in 1 cup water for 10 minutes.

2. Strain and drink warm.

- *Dosage:* 1 cup daily

- *Caution:* Avoid excessive use.

243. Bay Bark (*Laurus nobilis*)

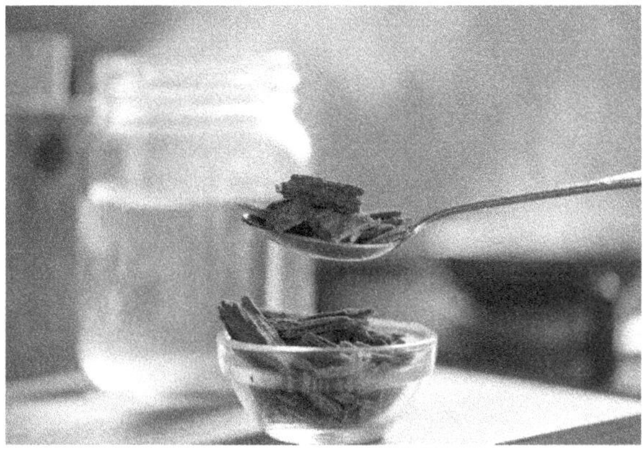

- *Part Used:* Bark

- *Traditional Uses:* Circulation, digestion

- *Preparation:*

1. Boil 1 teaspoon dried bark in 1 cup water for 10 minutes.

2. Strain and drink warm.

- *Dosage:* 1 cup daily

- *Caution:* Use moderately.

244. Red Maple Bark (*Acer rubrum*)

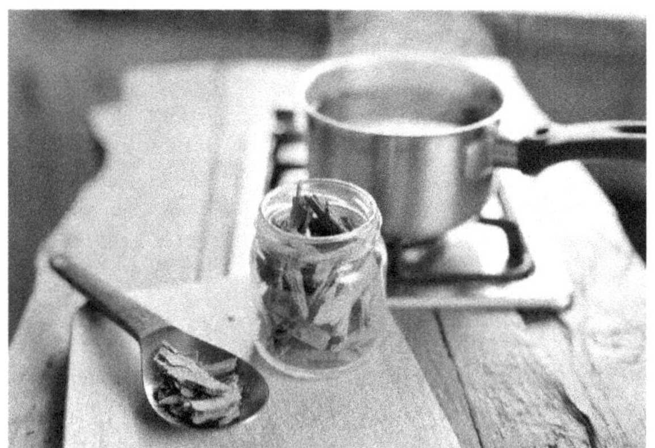

- *Part Used:* Bark

- *Traditional Uses:* Blood purifier, circulation

- *Preparation:*

1. Boil 1 tablespoon bark in 2 cups water for 20 minutes.

2. Strain and drink warm.

- *Dosage:* ½ cup twice daily

- *Caution:* Use cautiously.

245. Dogwood Bark (*Cornus florida*)

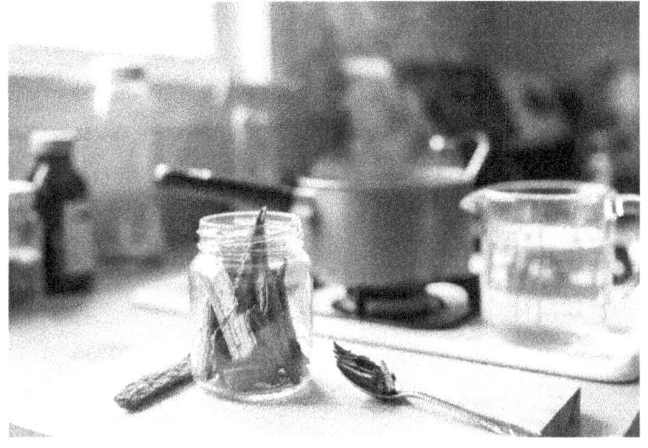

- *Part Used:* Bark

- *Traditional Uses:* Blood cleansing, circulation

- *Preparation:*

1. Boil 1 tablespoon dried bark in 2 cups water for 15 minutes.

2. Strain and drink warm.

- *Dosage:* ½ cup twice daily

- *Caution:* Moderate use advised.

246. Witch Hazel Bark (*Hamamelis virginiana*)

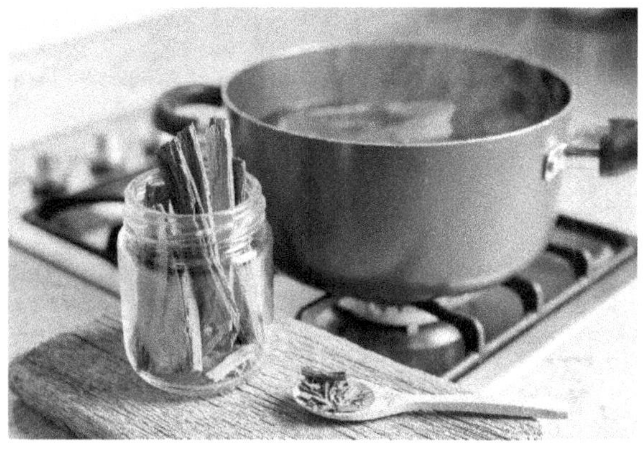

- *Part Used:* Bark

- *Traditional Uses:* Circulation, blood vessel support

- *Preparation:*

1. Boil 1 tablespoon bark in 2 cups water for 15 minutes.

2. Strain and drink warm or use externally.

- *Dosage:* ½ cup twice daily

- *Caution:* Avoid if allergic.

247. Black Walnut Bark (*Juglans nigra*)

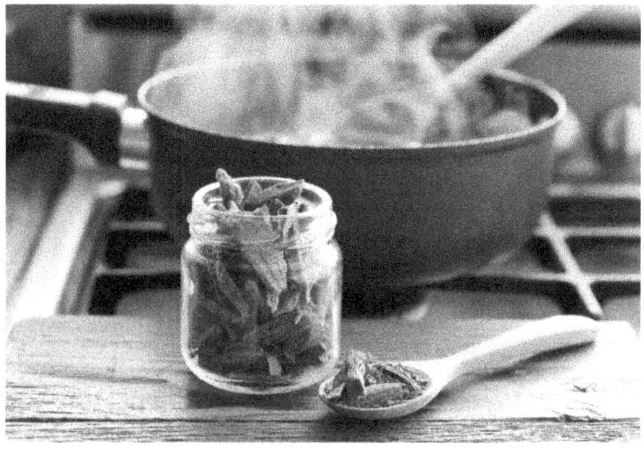

- *Part Used:* Bark

- *Traditional Uses:* Blood cleansing, parasitic infections

- *Preparation:*

1. Boil 1 tablespoon bark in 2 cups water for 15 minutes.

2. Strain and drink warm.

- *Dosage:* ½ cup twice daily

- *Caution:* Allergies possible.

248. Red Oak Bark (*Quercus rubra*)

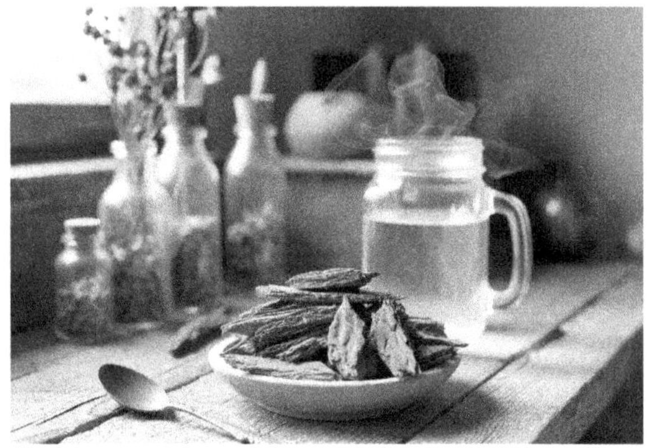

- ***Part Used:*** Bark

- ***Traditional Uses:*** Circulation, antimicrobial

- ***Preparation:***

1. Boil 1 tablespoon dried bark in 2 cups water for 15 minutes.

2. Strain and drink or use externally.

- ***Dosage:*** ½ cup twice daily

- ***Caution:*** Avoid prolonged use.

249. Yellow Birch Bark (*Betula alleghaniensis*)

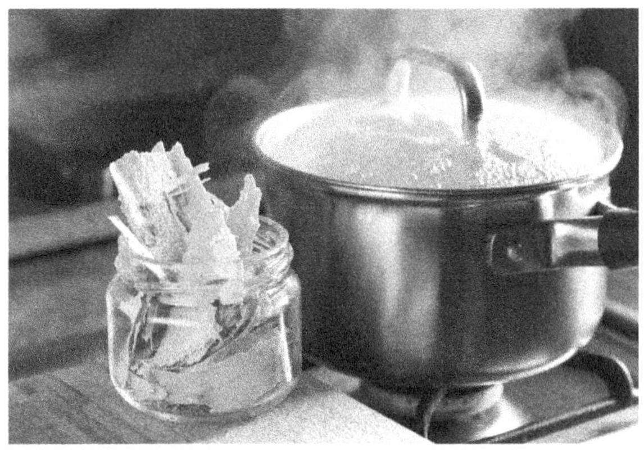

- *Part Used:* Bark

- *Traditional Uses:* Anti-inflammatory, circulation

- *Preparation:*

1. Boil 1 tablespoon bark in 2 cups water for 15 minutes.

2. Strain and drink warm.

- *Dosage:* 1 cup daily

- *Caution:* Allergies possible.

250. Bay Bark (*Laurus nobilis*)

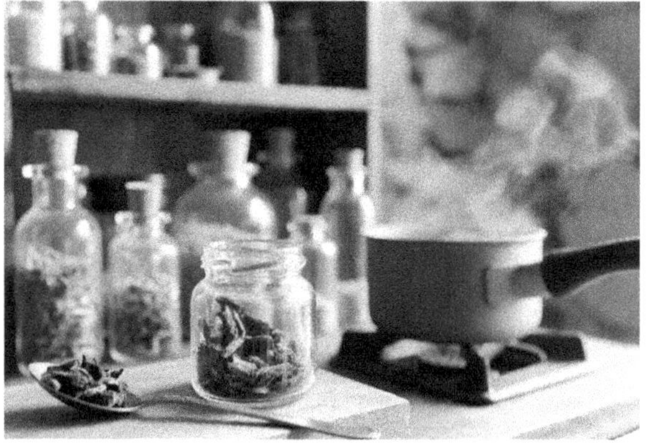

- *Part Used:* Bark

- *Traditional Uses:* Circulation, digestion support

- *Preparation:*

1. Boil 1 teaspoon dried bark in 1 cup water for 10 minutes.

2. Strain and drink warm.

- *Dosage:* 1 cup daily

- *Caution:* Avoid large doses.

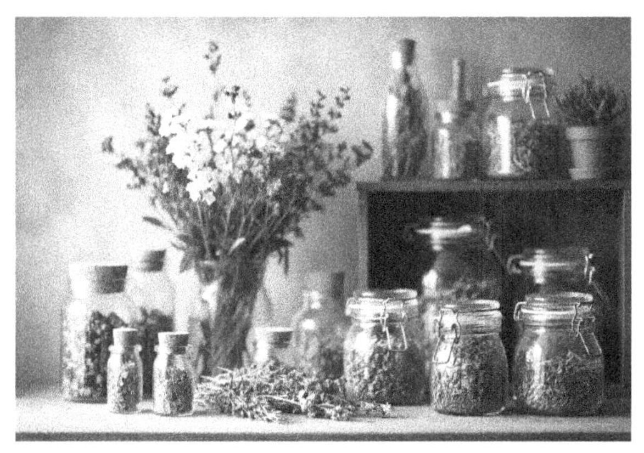

SECTION V: FLOWERS & AROMATIC HERBS

(Remedies 251–300)

*Mental Wellness, Anxiety &
Mood-support Flowers (251-270)*

251. Passionflower (*Passiflora incarnata*)

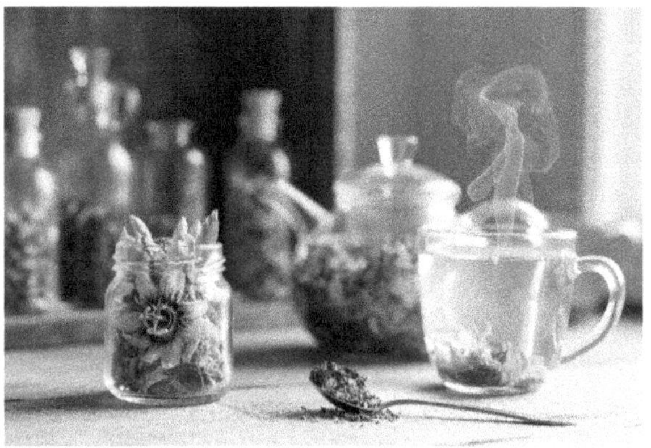

- *Part Used:* Flowers and leaves

- *Traditional Uses:* Anxiety, insomnia, nervous tension

- *Preparation:*

1. Add 1 teaspoon dried flowers and leaves to 1 cup boiling water.

2. Cover and steep for 10–15 minutes.

3. Strain and drink warm.

- *Dosage:* 1 cup 1–2 times daily

- *Caution:* May cause drowsiness; avoid combining with sedatives.

252. Lavender (*Lavandula angustifolia*)

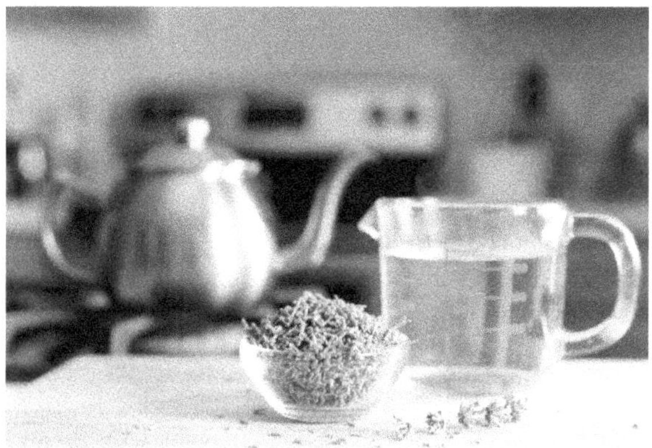

- *Part Used:* Flowers

- *Traditional Uses:* Anxiety, insomnia, mood elevation

- *Preparation:*

1. Add 1 teaspoon dried lavender flowers to 1 cup boiling water.

2. Steep covered for 10 minutes.

3. Strain and drink warm.

- *Dosage:* 1 cup up to twice daily

- *Caution:* Allergic reactions possible in sensitive individuals.

253. Chamomile (*Matricaria chamomilla*)

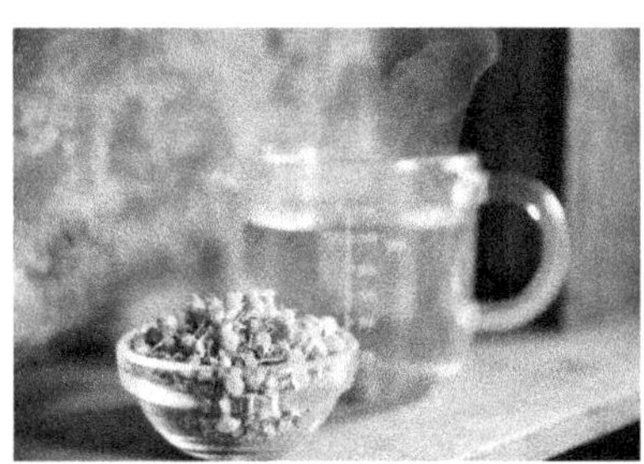

- *Part Used:* Flowers

- *Traditional Uses:* Sleep aid, anxiety, digestive relaxation

- *Preparation:*

1. Add 1 teaspoon dried chamomile flowers to 1 cup boiling water.

2. Cover and steep for 10 minutes.

3. Strain and drink warm, preferably before bedtime.

- *Dosage:* 1 cup at night

- *Caution:* Avoid if allergic to ragweed or related plants.

254. Lemon Balm (*Melissa officinalis*)

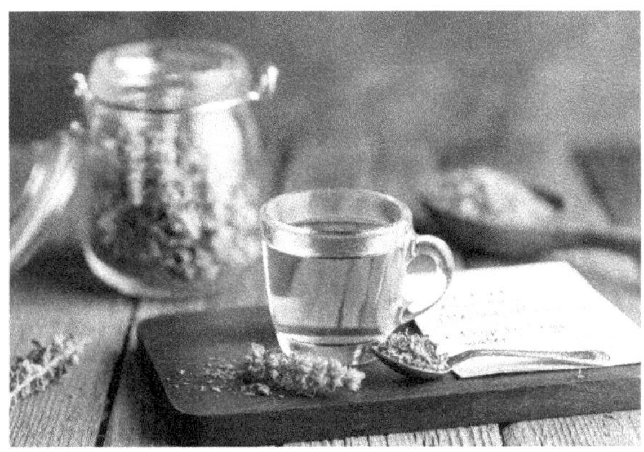

- *Part Used:* Leaves and flowers

- *Traditional Uses:* Anxiety, mood elevation, mild sedation

- *Preparation:*

1. Add 1 teaspoon dried lemon balm leaves and flowers to 1 cup boiling water.

2. Steep for 10 minutes.

3. Strain and drink warm.

- *Dosage:* 1–2 cups daily

- *Caution:* Generally safe; avoid high doses in pregnancy.

255. Valerian (*Valeriana officinalis*)

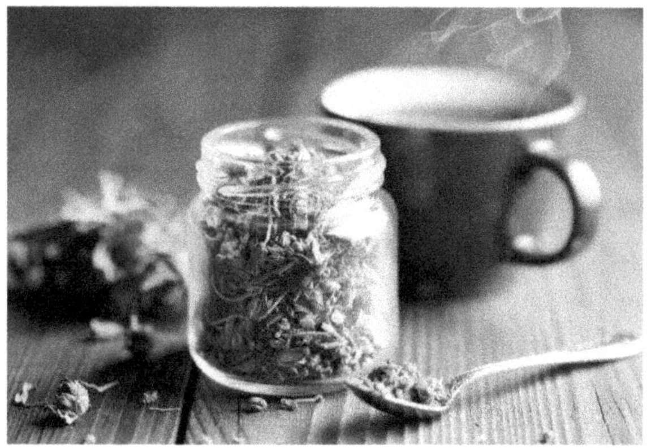

- *Part Used:* Flowers and roots

- *Traditional Uses:* Insomnia, anxiety, muscle relaxation

- *Preparation:*

1. Add 1 teaspoon dried flowers or root to 1 cup boiling water.

2. Cover and steep for 10–15 minutes.

3. Strain and drink warm.

- *Dosage:* 1 cup at night

- *Caution:* May cause drowsiness; avoid mixing with alcohol or sedatives.

256. Rose (*Rosa damascena*)

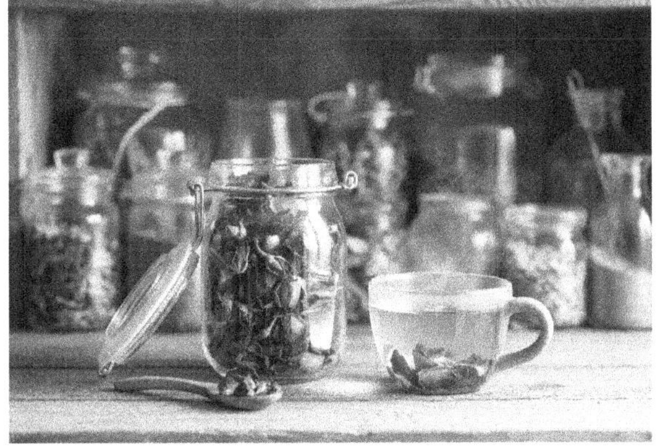

- *Part Used:* Petals

- *Traditional Uses:* Mood enhancement, anxiety relief

- *Preparation:*

1. Add 1 tablespoon fresh or 1 teaspoon dried rose petals to 1 cup boiling water.

2. Steep for 10 minutes.

3. Strain and drink warm.

- *Dosage:* 1 cup daily

- *Caution:* Generally safe.

257. Jasmine (*Jasminum sambac*)

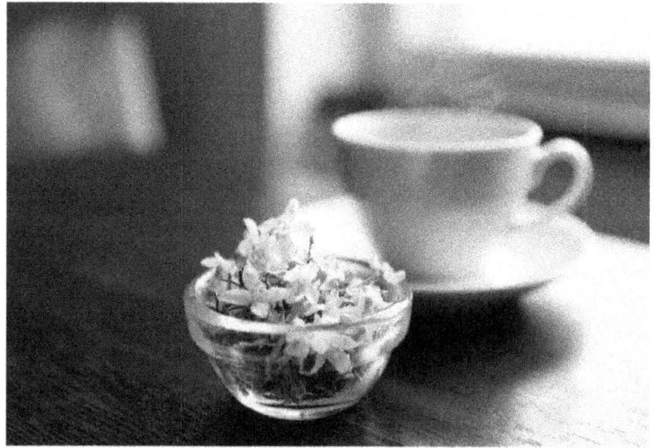

- *Part Used:* Flowers

- *Traditional Uses:* Stress relief, mood booster

- *Preparation:*

1. Add 1 teaspoon dried jasmine flowers to 1 cup boiling water.

2. Cover and steep for 10 minutes.

3. Strain and drink warm.

- *Dosage:* 1 cup daily

- *Caution:* Use moderately.

258. Hibiscus (*Hibiscus sabdariffa*)

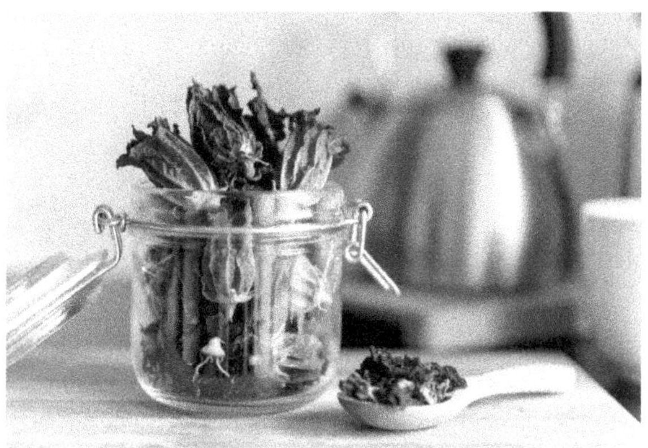

- ***Part Used:*** Flowers (calyces)

- ***Traditional Uses:*** Stress relief, blood pressure support

- ***Preparation:***

1. Add 1 tablespoon dried hibiscus calyces to 1 cup boiling water.

2. Steep for 10 minutes.

3. Strain and drink warm or cold.

- ***Dosage:*** 1–2 cups daily

- ***Caution:*** May lower blood pressure; avoid if hypotensive.

259. Marigold (*Calendula officinalis*)

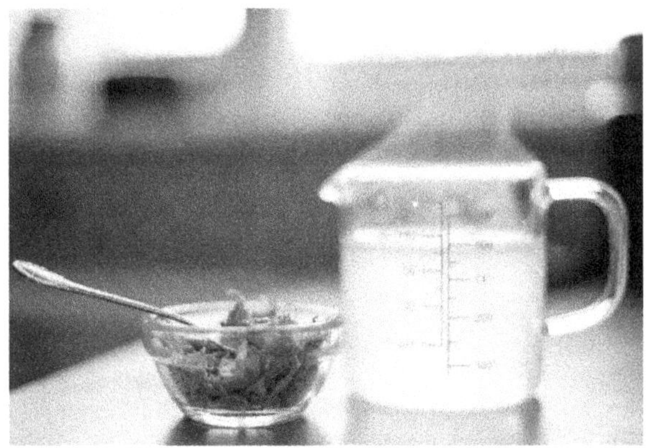

- *Part Used:* Flowers

- *Traditional Uses:* Mood support, anti-inflammatory

- *Preparation:*

1. Add 1 teaspoon dried marigold flowers to 1 cup boiling water.

2. Steep for 10 minutes.

3. Strain and drink warm.

- *Dosage:* 1 cup daily

- *Caution:* Allergies possible.

260. Chrysanthemum (*Chrysanthemum morifolium*)

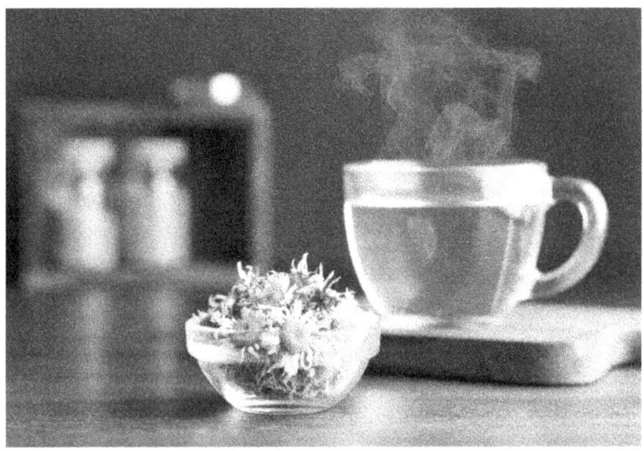

- *Part Used:* Flowers

- *Traditional Uses:* Calmative, anxiety relief

- *Preparation:*

1. Add 1 teaspoon dried chrysanthemum flowers to 1 cup boiling water.

2. Cover and steep for 10 minutes.

3. Strain and drink warm.

- *Dosage:* 1–2 cups daily

- *Caution:* Avoid in cases of cold or flu with fever.

261. Linden Flower (*Tilia cordata*)

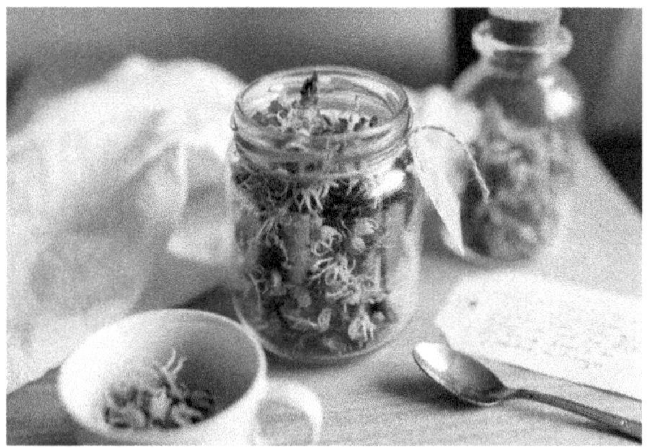

- ***Part Used:*** Flowers

- ***Traditional Uses:*** Anxiety, insomnia, nervous tension

- ***Preparation:***

1. Add 1 tablespoon dried linden flowers to 1 cup boiling water.

2. Cover and steep for 15 minutes.

3. Strain and drink warm.

- ***Dosage:*** 1 cup 1–2 times daily

- ***Caution:*** Generally safe.

262. Elderflower (*Sambucus nigra*)

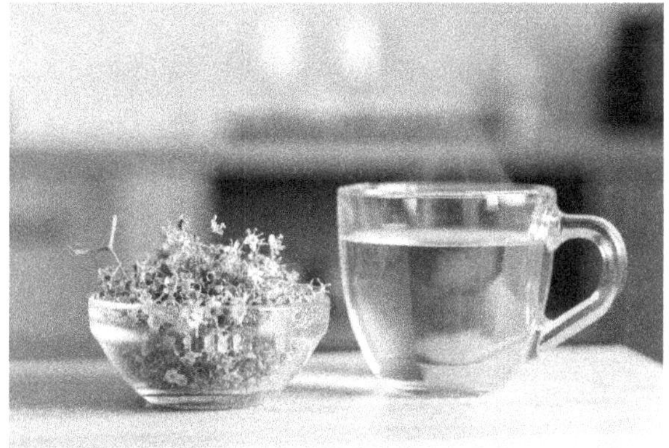

- *Part Used:* Flowers

- *Traditional Uses:* Mood support, immune boost

- *Preparation:*

1. Add 1 tablespoon dried elderflowers to 1 cup boiling water.

2. Steep for 10 minutes.

3. Strain and drink warm.

- *Dosage:* 1 cup daily

- *Caution:* Avoid raw berries; toxic if unprepared.

263. Blue Lotus (*Nymphaea caerulea*)

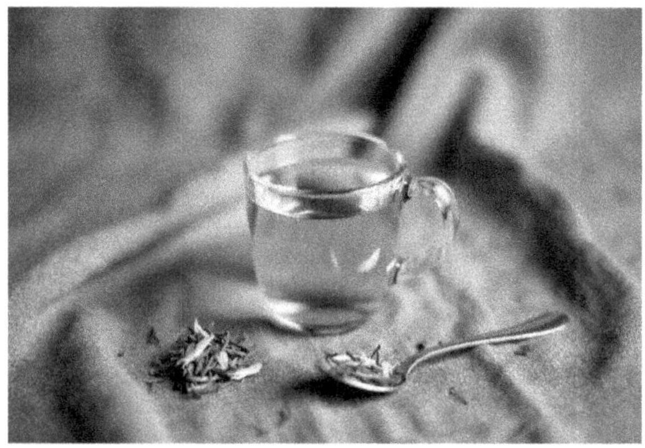

- *Part Used:* Flowers

- *Traditional Uses:* Relaxation, mild euphoria, anxiety relief

- *Preparation:*

1. Add 1 teaspoon dried blue lotus flowers to 1 cup hot water (not boiling).

2. Steep for 15 minutes.

3. Strain and drink warm.

- *Dosage:* 1 cup daily

- *Caution:* Avoid in pregnancy and with sedatives.

264. Sweet Violet (*Viola odorata*)

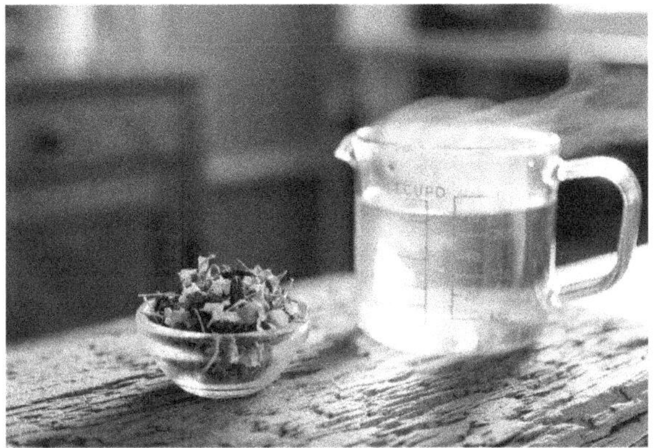

- *Part Used:* Flowers

- *Traditional Uses:* Mood enhancer, mild sedative

- *Preparation:*

1. Add 1 teaspoon dried violet flowers to 1 cup boiling water.

2. Steep for 10 minutes.

3. Strain and drink warm.

- *Dosage:* 1 cup daily

- *Caution:* Generally safe.

265. Yarrow (*Achillea millefolium*)

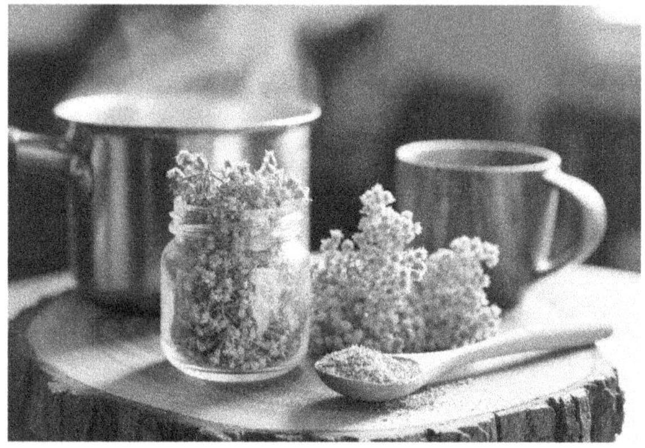

- *Part Used:* Flowers

- *Traditional Uses:* Anxiety, stress relief

- *Preparation:*

1. Add 1 teaspoon dried yarrow flowers to 1 cup boiling water.

2. Steep for 10 minutes.

3. Strain and drink warm.

- *Dosage:* 1 cup daily

- *Caution:* Avoid if allergic to ragweed.

266. Magnolia (*Magnolia officinalis*)

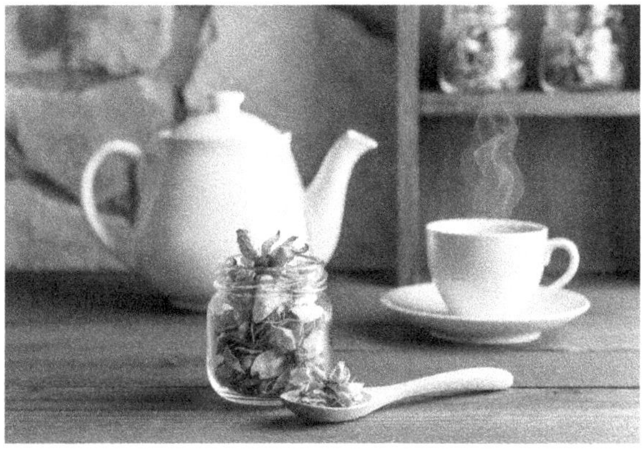

- *Part Used:* Flowers and bark

- *Traditional Uses:* Anxiety, stress relief

- *Preparation:*

1. Add 1 teaspoon dried magnolia flowers to 1 cup boiling water.

2. Steep for 10–15 minutes.

3. Strain and drink warm.

- *Dosage:* 1 cup daily

- *Caution:* Avoid in pregnancy.

267. Elderberry Flowers (*Sambucus nigra*)

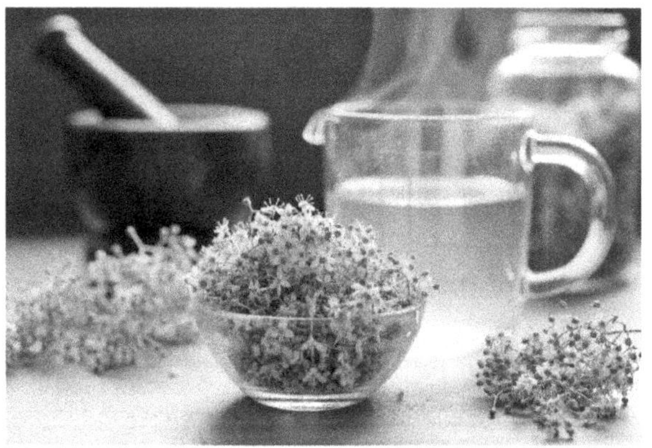

- *Part Used:* Flowers

- *Traditional Uses:* Mood support, immune system

- *Preparation:*

1. Add 1 tablespoon dried elderflowers to 1 cup boiling water.

2. Steep for 10 minutes.

3. Strain and drink warm.

- *Dosage:* 1 cup daily

- *Caution:* Avoid raw berries.

268. Calendula (*Calendula officinalis*)

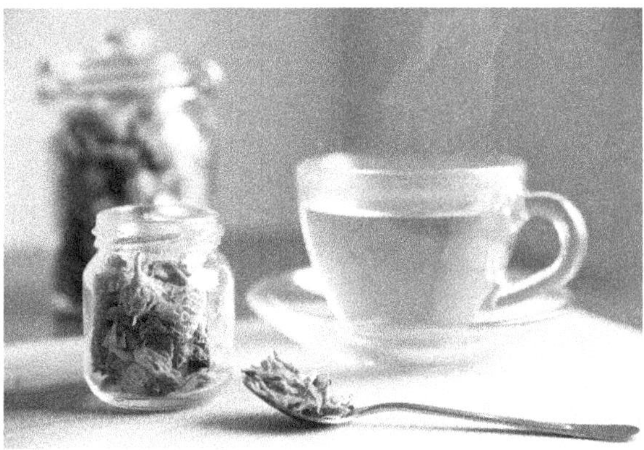

- ***Part Used:*** Flowers

- ***Traditional Uses:*** Anti-inflammatory, mood support

- ***Preparation:***

1. Add 1 teaspoon dried calendula flowers to 1 cup boiling water.

2. Steep for 10 minutes.

3. Strain and drink warm.

- ***Dosage:*** 1 cup daily

- ***Caution:*** Avoid if allergic to daisies.

269. Rosehip Flowers (*Rosa canina*)

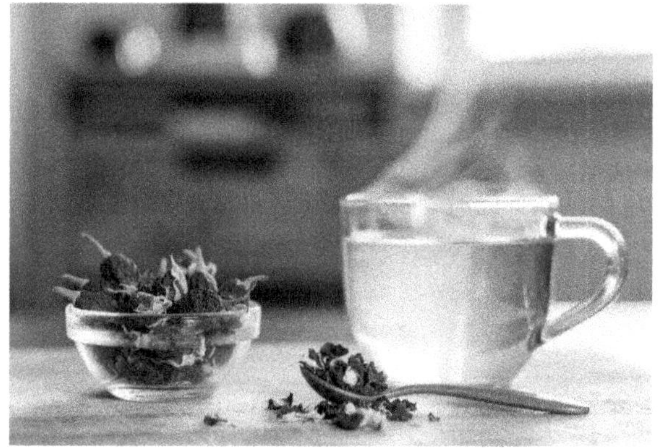

- *Part Used:* Flowers and hips

- *Traditional Uses:* Mood enhancer, vitamin C source

- *Preparation:*

1. Add 1 teaspoon dried rosehips and flowers to 1 cup boiling water.

2. Steep for 15 minutes.

3. Strain and drink warm.

- *Dosage:* 1 cup daily

- *Caution:* Generally safe.

270. Jasmine Flowers (*Jasminum sambac*)

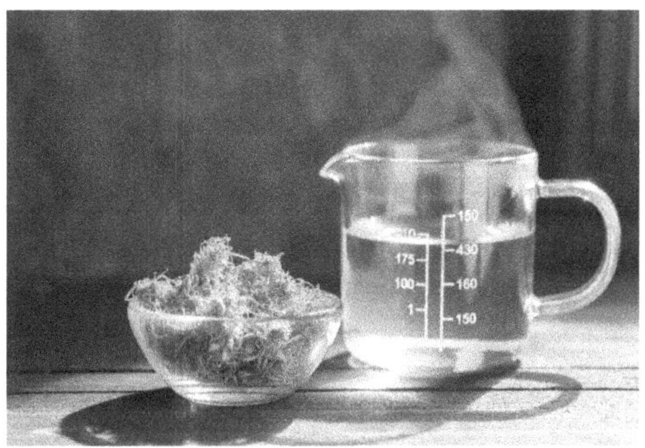

- *Part Used:* Flowers

- *Traditional Uses:* Stress relief, mood booster

- *Preparation:*

1. Add 1 teaspoon dried jasmine flowers to 1 cup boiling water.

2. Steep for 10 minutes.

3. Strain and drink warm.

- *Dosage:* 1 cup daily

- *Caution:* Use moderately.

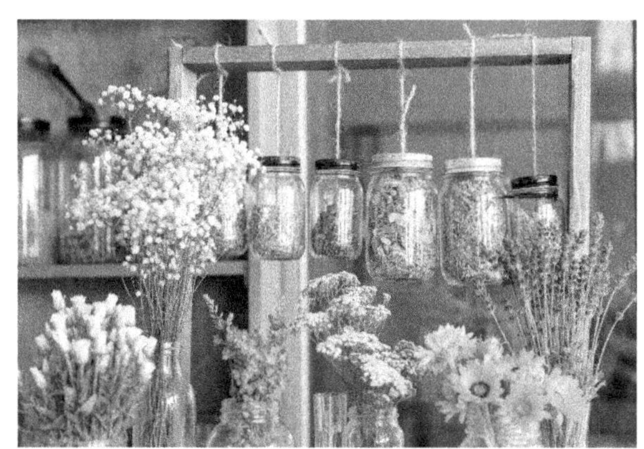

Skin, Beauty, Wound-healing & Anti-aging Flowers (271-300)

271. Calendula (*Calendula officinalis*)

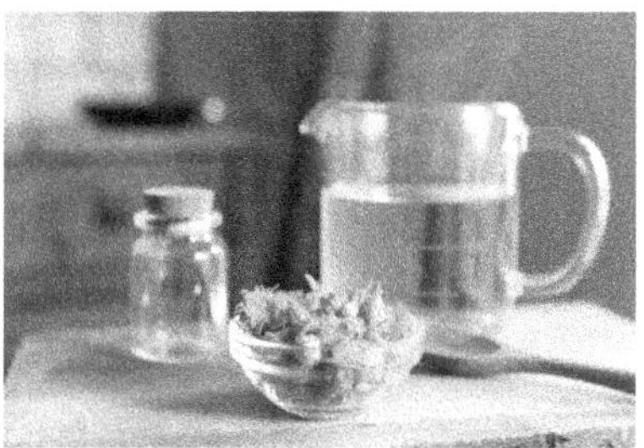

- *Part Used:* Flowers

- *Traditional Uses:* Wound healing, skin inflammation, anti-aging

- *Preparation:*

1. Add 1 tablespoon dried calendula flowers to 1 cup boiling water.

2. Steep for 10–15 minutes.

3. Strain and use as a wash or drink as tea for skin support.

- *Dosage:* Apply externally or drink 1 cup daily

- *Caution:* Avoid if allergic to daisies or chrysanthemums.

272. Chamomile (*Matricaria chamomilla*)

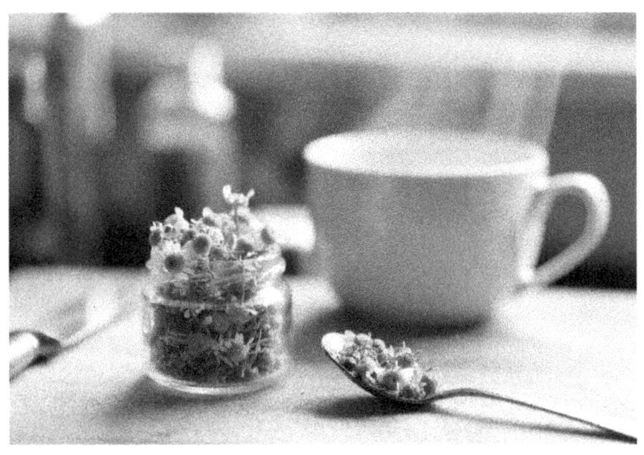

- *Part Used:* Flowers

- *Traditional Uses:* Skin irritation, acne, anti-inflammatory

- *Preparation:*

1. Steep 1 tablespoon dried chamomile flowers in 1 cup boiling water for 10 minutes.

2. Strain and use as facial wash or compress.

- *Dosage:* Apply externally or drink 1 cup daily

- *Caution:* Avoid if allergic to ragweed.

273. Rose (*Rosa damascena*)

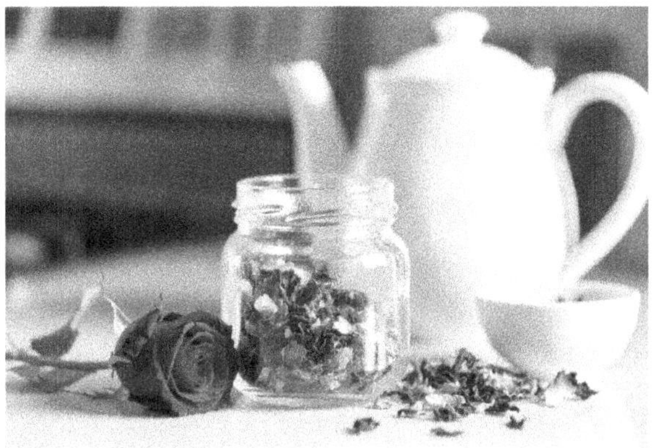

- ***Part Used:*** Petals

- ***Traditional Uses:*** Skin hydration, anti-aging, soothing

- ***Preparation:***

1. Steep 1 tablespoon fresh or dried rose petals in 1 cup boiling water for 10 minutes.

2. Strain and use as toner or drink as tea.

- ***Dosage:*** Apply topically or drink 1 cup daily

- ***Caution:*** Generally safe.

274. Lavender (*Lavandula angustifolia*)

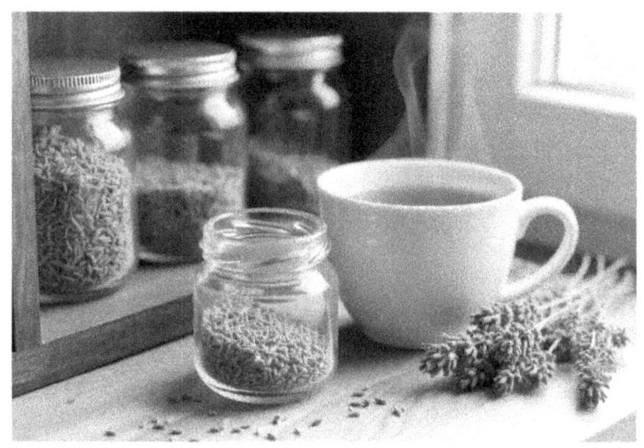

- *Part Used:* Flowers

- *Traditional Uses:* Skin healing, acne, anti-inflammatory

- *Preparation:*

1. Steep 1 teaspoon dried lavender flowers in 1 cup boiling water for 10 minutes.

2. Strain and apply as compress or use tea internally.

- *Dosage:* Use externally or drink 1 cup daily

- *Caution:* Allergic reactions possible.

275. Hibiscus (*Hibiscus sabdariffa*)

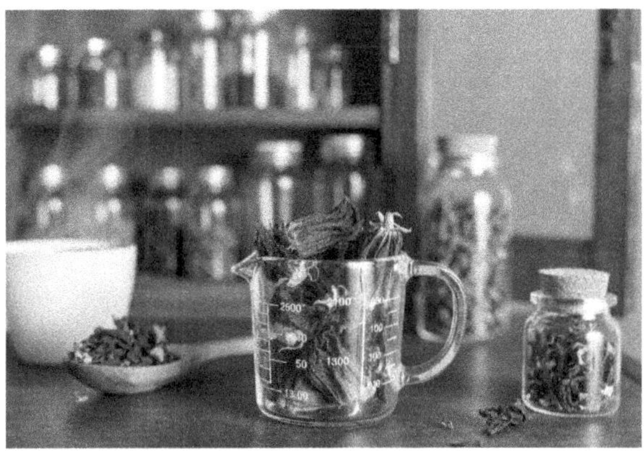

- *Part Used:* Flowers (calyces)

- *Traditional Uses:* Skin toning, anti-aging, antioxidant

- *Preparation:*

1. Steep 1 tablespoon dried hibiscus calyces in 1 cup boiling water for 10 minutes.

2. Strain and use as facial rinse or drink.

- *Dosage:* Apply externally or drink 1–2 cups daily

- *Caution:* May lower blood pressure.

276. Aloe Vera (*Aloe barbadensis*)

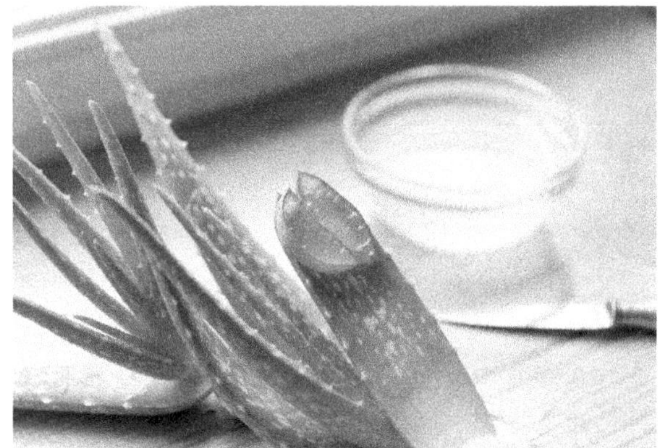

- *Part Used:* Gel

- *Traditional Uses:* Skin hydration, burns, anti-inflammatory

- *Preparation:*

1. Extract fresh gel from leaves.

2. Apply directly to skin or mix with other ingredients for topical use.

- *Dosage:* Apply externally as needed

- *Caution:* Avoid oral use long-term.

277. Calendula (*Calendula officinalis*)

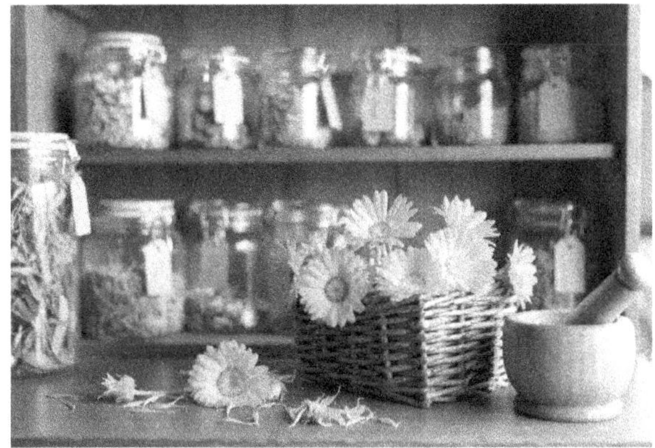

- *Part Used:* Flowers

- *Traditional Uses:* Anti-inflammatory, wound healing

- *Preparation:*

1. Prepare infusion as above.

2. Use as compress or wash.

- *Dosage:* External use

- *Caution:* Allergy to daisies.

278. Witch Hazel (*Hamamelis virginiana*)

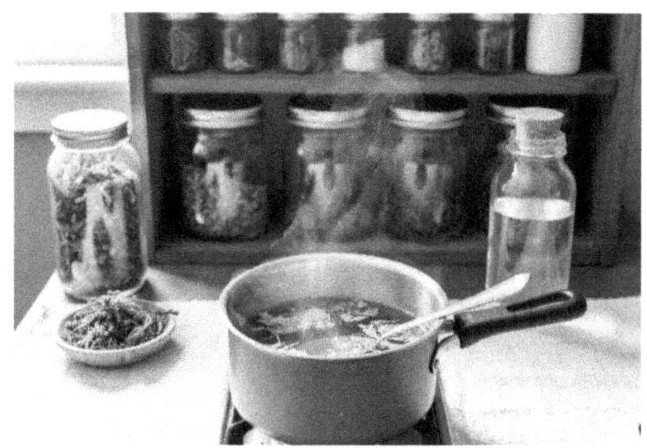

- *Part Used:* Bark and leaves

- *Traditional Uses:* Skin tightening, anti-inflammatory

- *Preparation:*

1. Boil 1 tablespoon dried leaves or bark in 2 cups water for 15 minutes.

2. Strain and use as toner.

- *Dosage:* External use

- *Caution:* Avoid internal use.

279. Yarrow (*Achillea millefolium*)

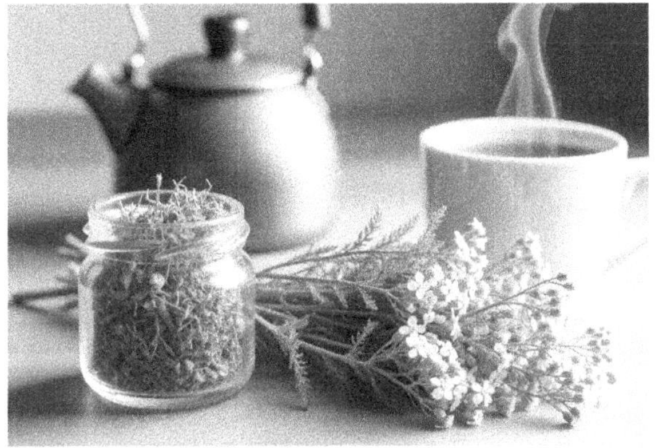

- *Part Used:* Flowers

- *Traditional Uses:* Wound healing, anti-inflammatory

- *Preparation:*

1. Steep 1 teaspoon dried flowers in 1 cup boiling water for 10 minutes.

2. Strain and use as compress or wash.

- *Dosage:* External use

- *Caution:* Allergy risk.

280. Rosehip (*Rosa canina*)

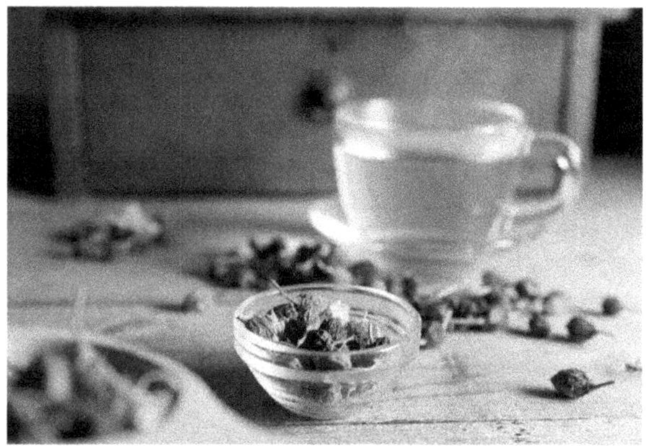

- *Part Used:* Fruits and flowers

- *Traditional Uses:* Skin regeneration, anti-aging, vitamin C source

- *Preparation:*

1. Steep 1 teaspoon dried rosehips and flowers in 1 cup boiling water for 15 minutes.

2. Strain and drink or apply topically.

- *Dosage:* 1 cup daily or topical use

- *Caution:* Generally safe.

281. Gotu Kola (*Centella asiatica*)

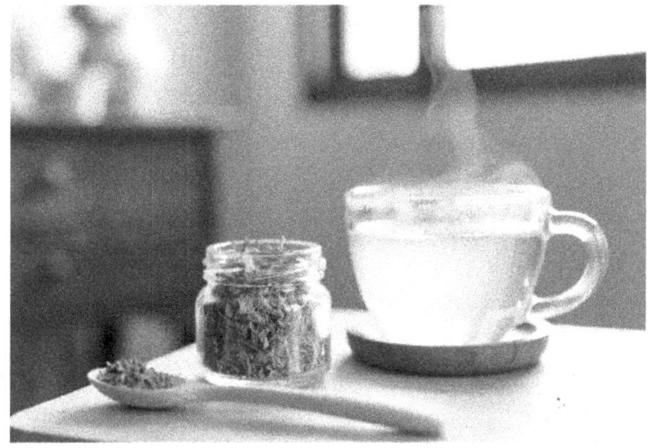

- *Part Used:* Leaves and flowers

- *Traditional Uses:* Skin healing, collagen production

- *Preparation:*

1. Steep 1 teaspoon dried leaves in 1 cup boiling water for 10 minutes.

2. Strain and drink or apply externally.

- *Dosage:* 1 cup daily or topical use

- *Caution:* Use cautiously in pregnancy.

282. Calendula (*Calendula officinalis*)

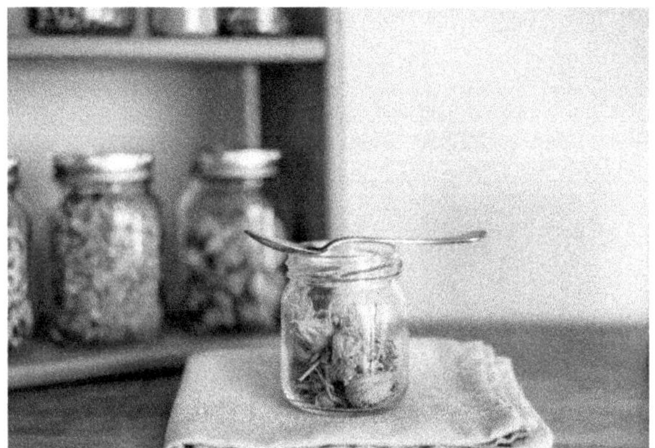

- ***Part Used:*** Flowers

- ***Traditional Uses:*** Anti-inflammatory, skin healing

- ***Preparation:***

1. Infuse as above.

2. Use externally as needed.

- ***Dosage:*** External use

- ***Caution:*** Allergy possible.

283. Chamomile (*Matricaria chamomilla*)

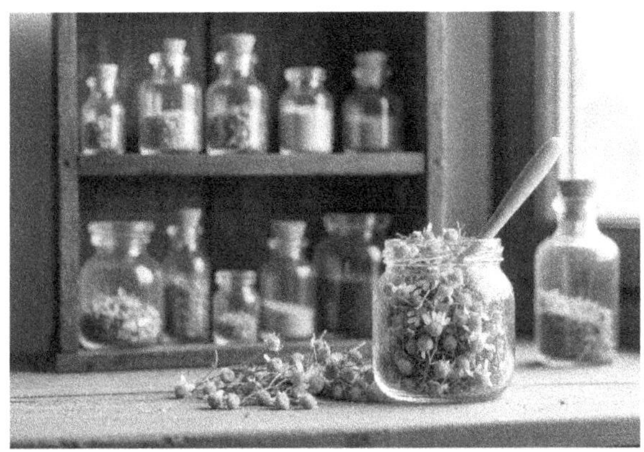

- *Part Used:* Flowers

- *Traditional Uses:* Skin calming, anti-inflammatory

- *Preparation:*

1. Prepare infusion as above.

2. Use topically or drink.

- *Dosage:* External or internal

- *Caution:* Allergy possible.

284. Lavender (*Lavandula angustifolia*)

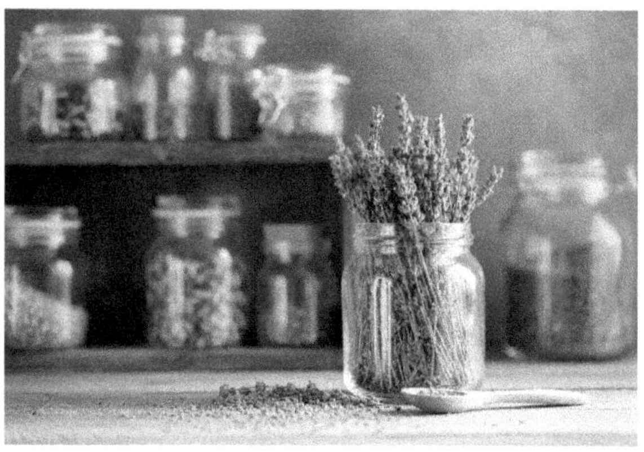

- ***Part Used:*** Flowers

- ***Traditional Uses:*** Skin healing, anti-inflammatory

- ***Preparation:***

1. Prepare infusion as above.

2. Use externally or drink.

- ***Dosage:*** External or internal

- ***Caution:*** Allergy possible.

285. Aloe Vera (*Aloe barbadensis*)

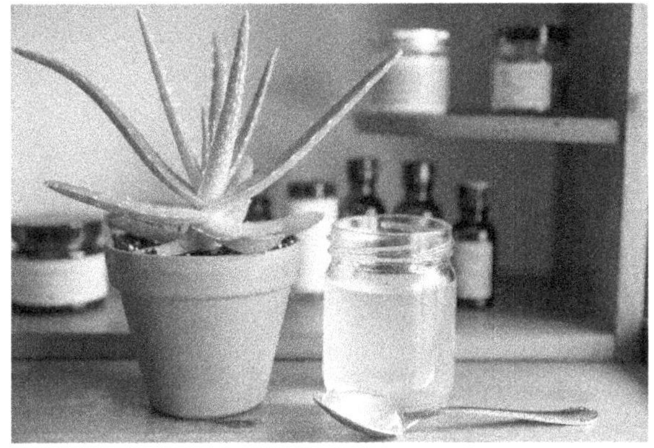

- *Part Used:* Gel

- *Traditional Uses:* Burns, skin hydration

- *Preparation:*

1. Extract fresh gel.

2. Apply externally.

- *Dosage:* External use

- *Caution:* Avoid oral use long-term.

286. Calendula (*Calendula officinalis*)

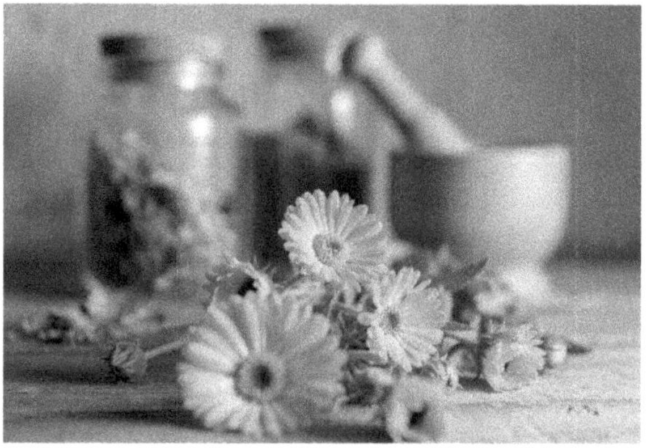

- *Part Used:* Flowers
- *Traditional Uses:* Wound healing
- *Preparation:*

1. Infuse as above.
2. Use externally.

- *Dosage:* External use
- *Caution:* Allergy possible.

287. Witch Hazel (*Hamamelis virginiana*)

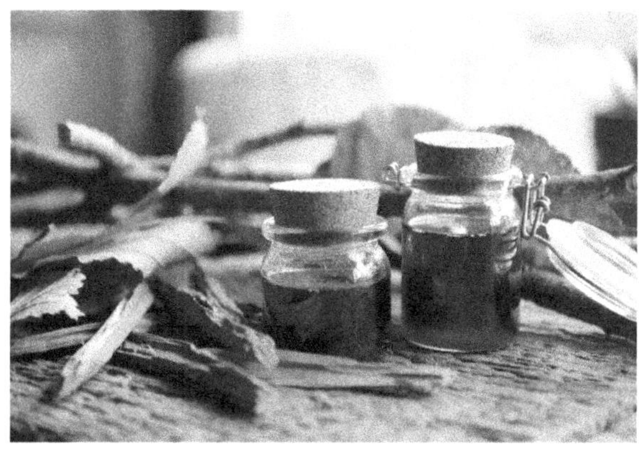

- *Part Used:* Bark and leaves

- *Traditional Uses:* Skin tightening, anti-inflammatory

- *Preparation:*

1. Prepare decoction as above.

2. Use as toner.

- **Dosage:** External use

- *Caution:* Avoid internal use.

288. Yarrow (*Achillea millefolium*)

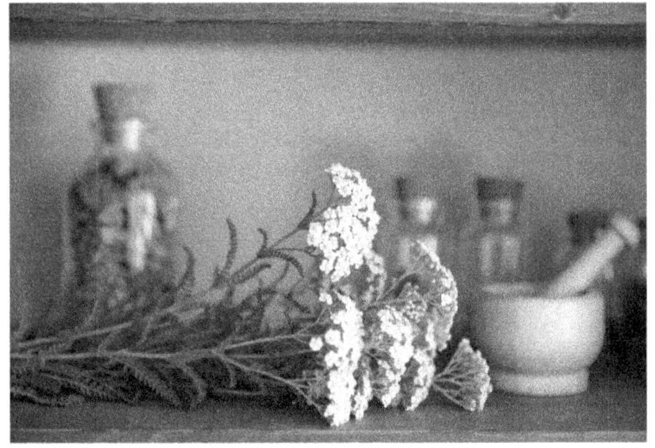

- *Part Used:* Flowers

- *Traditional Uses:* Wound healing

- *Preparation:*

1. Prepare infusion as above.

2. Use externally.

- *Dosage:* External use

- *Caution:* Allergy possible.

289. Rosehip (*Rosa canina*)

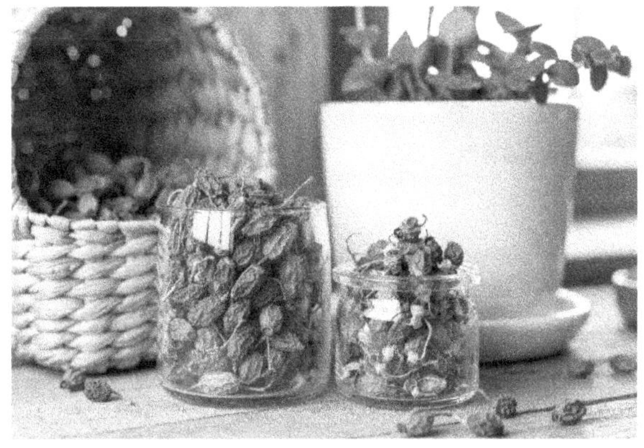

- *Part Used:* Fruits and flowers

- *Traditional Uses:* Skin rejuvenation, vitamin C source

- *Preparation:*

1. Prepare infusion as above.

2. Drink or use topically.

- *Dosage:* 1 cup daily or topical use

- *Caution:* Generally safe.

290. Gotu Kola (*Centella asiatica*)

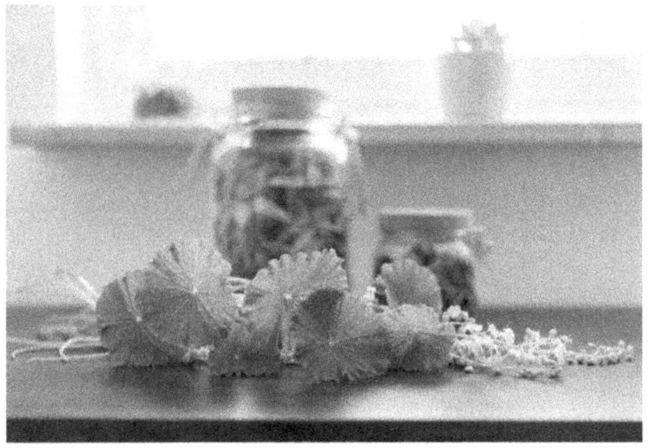

- *Part Used:* Leaves and flowers

- *Traditional Uses:* Skin healing, collagen production

- *Preparation:*

1. Prepare infusion as above.

2. Use externally or drink.

- *Dosage:* 1 cup daily or topical use

- *Caution:* Use cautiously in pregnancy.

291. Chamomile (*Matricaria chamomilla*)

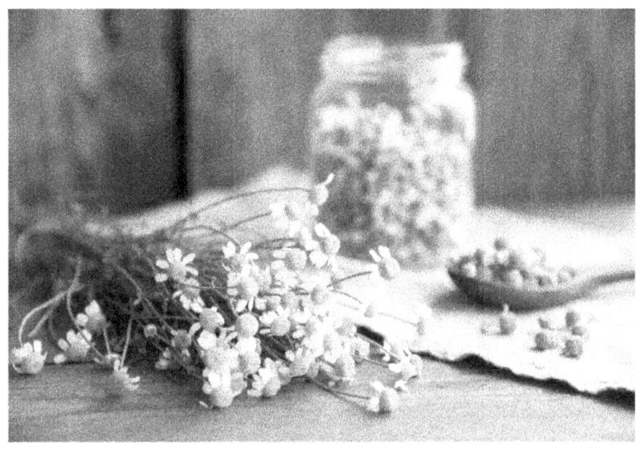

- *Part Used:* Flowers

- *Traditional Uses:* Skin calming

- *Preparation:*

1. Prepare infusion as above.

2. Use externally or drink.

- *Dosage:* External or internal

- *Caution:* Allergy possible.

292. Lavender (*Lavandula angustifolia*)

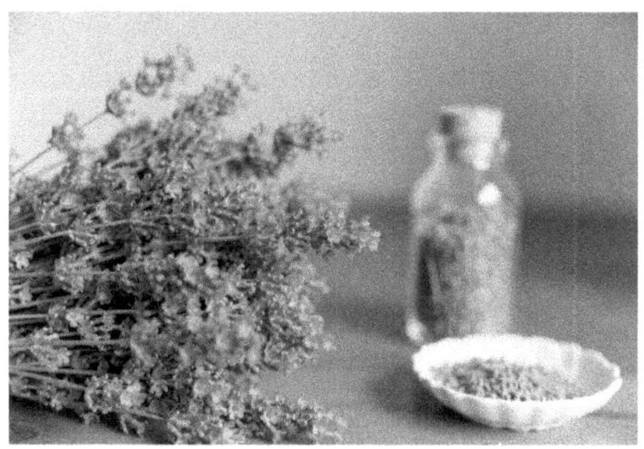

- *Part Used:* Flowers

- *Traditional Uses:* Skin healing

- *Preparation:*

1. Prepare infusion as above.

2. Use externally or drink.

- *Dosage:* External or internal

- *Caution:* Allergy possible.

293. Aloe Vera (*Aloe barbadensis*)

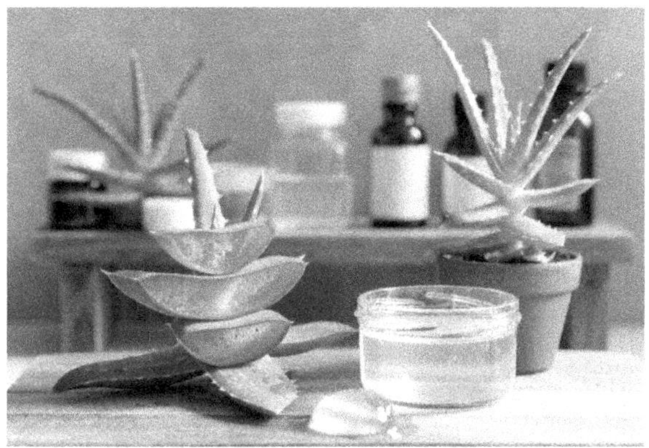

- *Part Used:* Gel

- *Traditional Uses:* Skin hydration, burns

- *Preparation:*

1. Extract fresh gel.

2. Apply externally.

- *Dosage:* External use

- *Caution:* Avoid oral use long-term.

294. Calendula (*Calendula officinalis*)

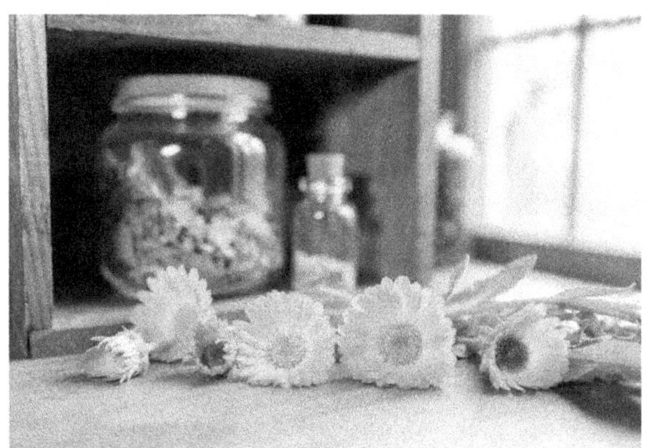

- ***Part Used:*** Flowers

- ***Traditional Uses:*** Anti-inflammatory, wound healing

- ***Preparation:***

1. Prepare infusion as above.

2. Use externally.

- ***Dosage:*** External use

- ***Caution:*** Allergy possible.

295. Witch Hazel (*Hamamelis virginiana*)

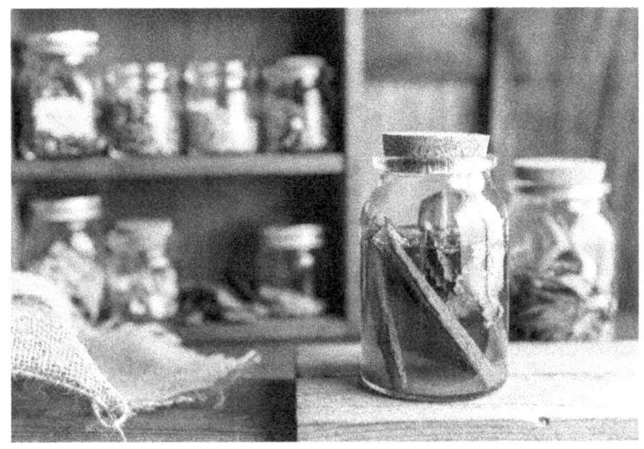

- ***Part Used:*** Bark and leaves

- ***Traditional Uses:*** Skin tightening

- ***Preparation:***

1. Prepare decoction as above.

2. Use as toner.

- ***Dosage:*** External use

- ***Caution:*** Avoid internal use.

296. Yarrow (*Achillea millefolium*)

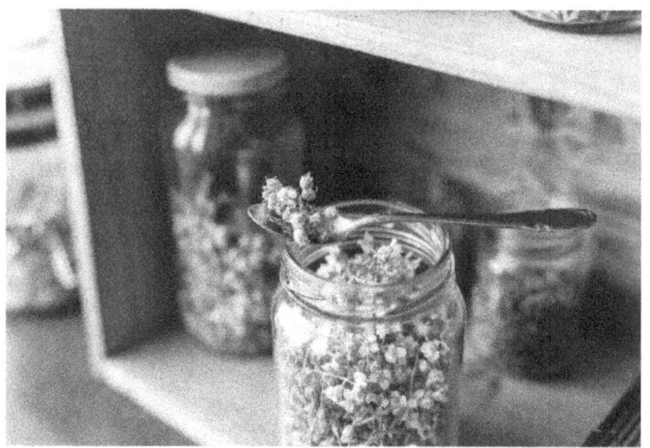

- ***Part Used:*** Flowers

- ***Traditional Uses:*** Wound healing

- ***Preparation:***

1. Prepare infusion as above.

2. Use externally.

- ***Dosage:*** External use

- ***Caution:*** Allergy possible.

297. Rosehip (*Rosa canina*)

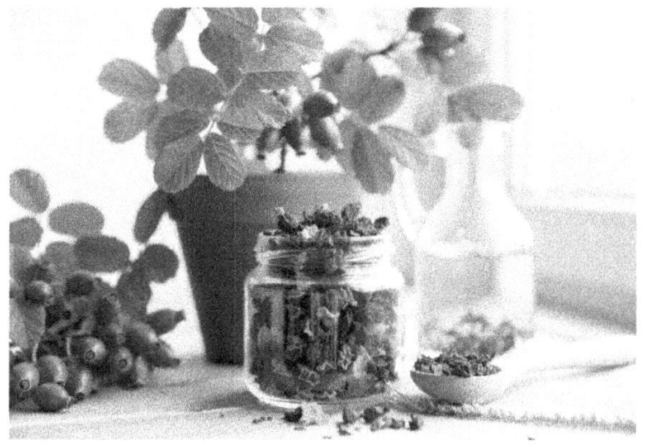

- *Part Used:* Fruits and flowers

- *Traditional Uses:* Skin rejuvenation

- *Preparation:*

1. Prepare infusion as above.

2. Use topically or drink.

- *Dosage:* 1 cup daily or topical use

- *Caution:* Generally safe.

298. Gotu Kola (*Centella asiatica*)

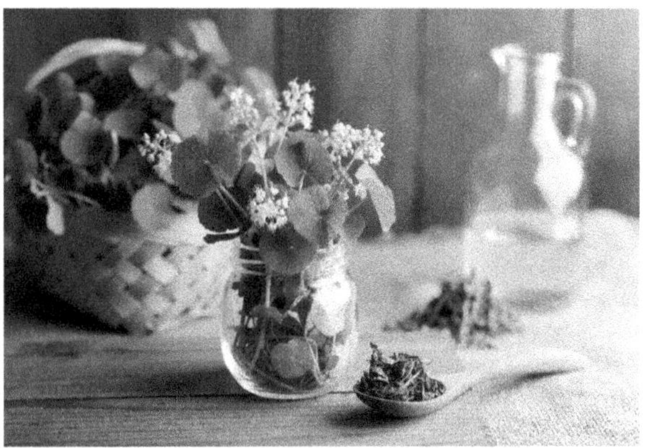

- *Part Used:* Leaves and flowers

- *Traditional Uses:* Skin healing

- *Preparation:*

1. Prepare infusion as above.

2. Use externally or drink.

- *Dosage:* 1 cup daily or topical use

- *Caution:* Use cautiously in pregnancy.

299. Chamomile (*Matricaria chamomilla*)

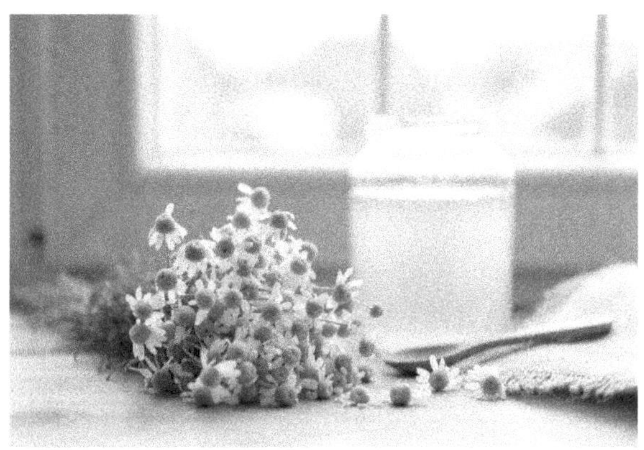

- *Part Used:* Flowers

- *Traditional Uses:* Skin calming

- *Preparation:*

1. Prepare infusion as above.

2. Use externally or drink.

- *Dosage:* External or internal

- *Caution:* Allergy possible.

300. Lavender (*Lavandula angustifolia*)

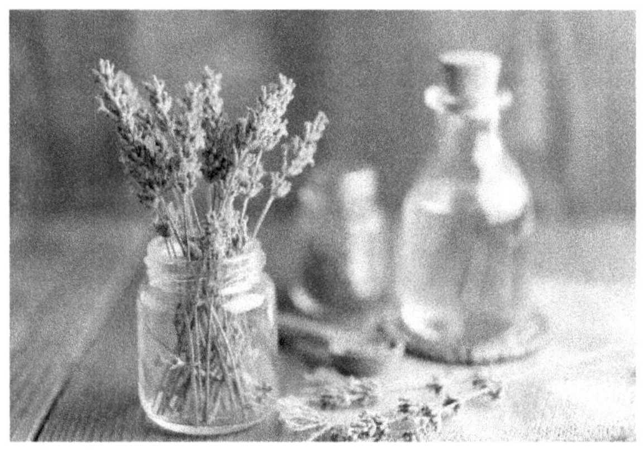

- *Part Used:* Flowers

- *Traditional Uses:* Skin healing

- *Preparation:*

1. Prepare infusion as above.

2. Use externally or drink.

- *Dosage:* External or internal

- *Caution:* Allergy possible.

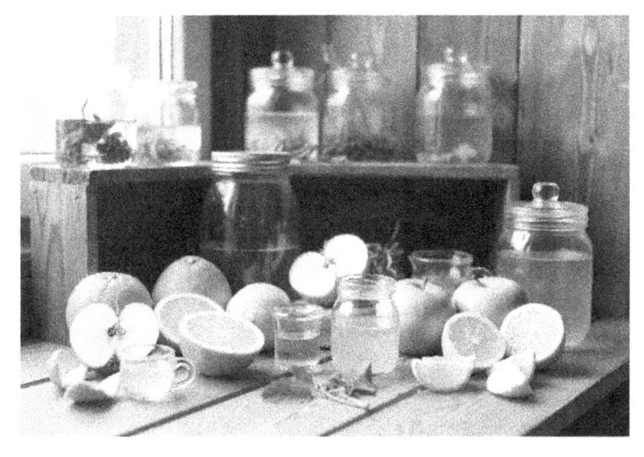

SECTION VI: FRUITS, PEELS & NATURAL EXTRACTS

(Remedies 301–350)

Immune-boosting, Vitamin-rich & Antioxidant Remedies (301-325)

301. Orange Peel (*Citrus sinensis*)

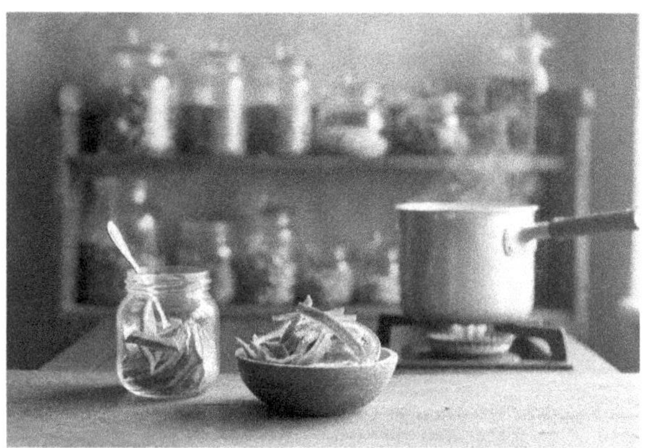

- *Part Used:* Peel

- **Traditional Uses:** Immune support, digestion, antioxidant

- *Preparation:*

1. Dry orange peel pieces thoroughly.

2. Boil 1 tablespoon dried peel in 2 cups water for 10 minutes.

3. Strain and drink warm as tea.

- *Dosage:* 1 cup daily

- *Caution:* Avoid if allergic to citrus.

302. Lemon Peel (*Citrus limon*)

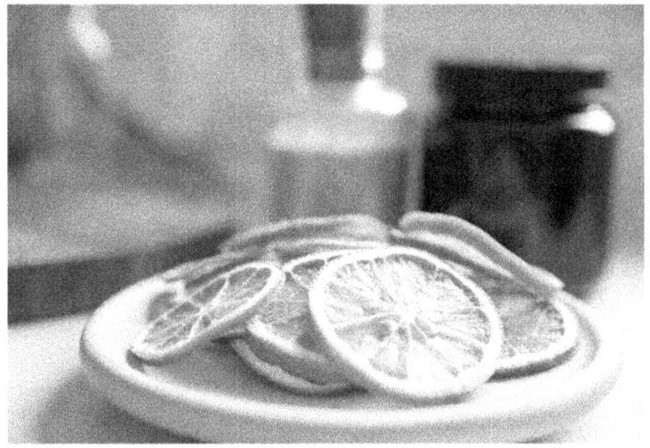

- ***Part Used:*** Peel

- ***Traditional Uses:*** Immunity, detox, antioxidant

- ***Preparation:***

1. Dry lemon peel and slice thinly.

2. Boil 1 tablespoon in 2 cups water for 10 minutes.

3. Strain and drink warm.

- ***Dosage:*** 1 cup daily

- ***Caution:*** Avoid excessive intake with sensitive stomach.

303. Pomegranate Peel (*Punica granatum*)

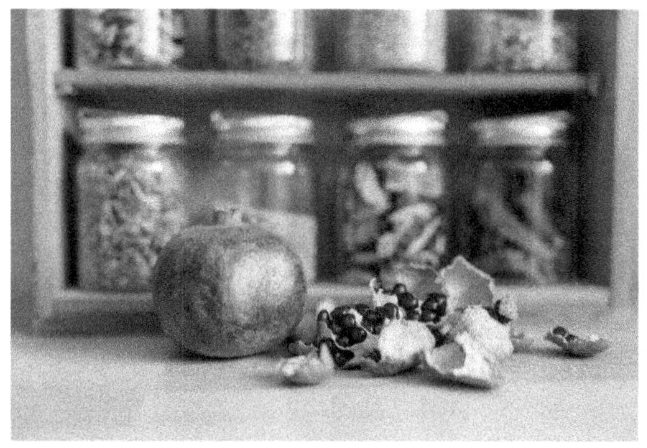

- *Part Used:* Peel

- *Traditional Uses:* Antioxidant, anti-inflammatory, immune boost

- *Preparation:*

1. Dry pomegranate peel pieces.

2. Boil 1 teaspoon dried peel in 2 cups water for 15 minutes.

3. Strain and drink warm.

- *Dosage:* 1 cup daily

- *Caution:* Use moderately.

304. Apple Peel (*Malus domestica*)

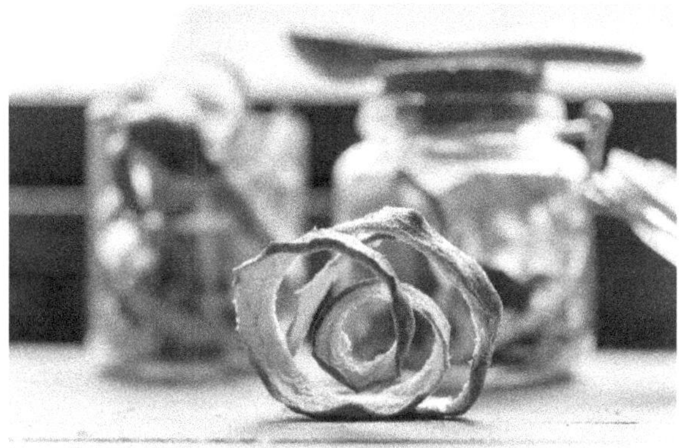

- *Part Used:* Peel

- *Traditional Uses:* Antioxidant, fiber source, immunity

- *Preparation:*

1. Wash and dry apple peels.

2. Steep 1 tablespoon dried peel in 1 cup hot water for 10 minutes.

3. Strain and drink.

- *Dosage:* 1 cup daily

- *Caution:* Use organic apples to avoid pesticides.

305. Grapefruit Peel (*Citrus paradisi*)

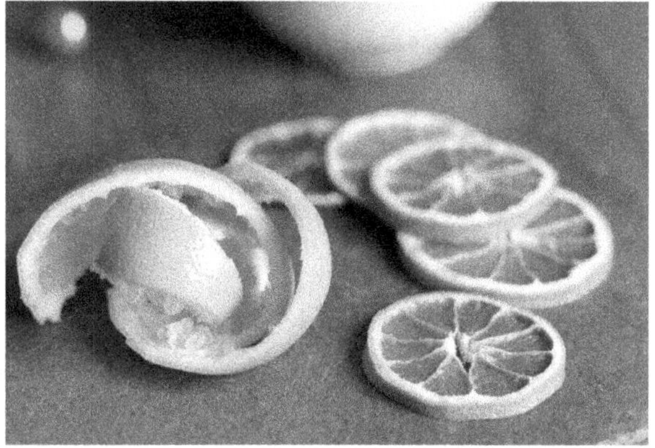

- *Part Used:* Peel

- *Traditional Uses:* Immunity, detox, antioxidant

- *Preparation:*

1. Dry grapefruit peel slices.

2. Boil 1 tablespoon in 2 cups water for 10 minutes.

3. Strain and drink warm.

- *Dosage:* 1 cup daily

- *Caution:* May interact with medications; consult doctor.

306. Acerola Cherry (*Malpighia emarginata*)

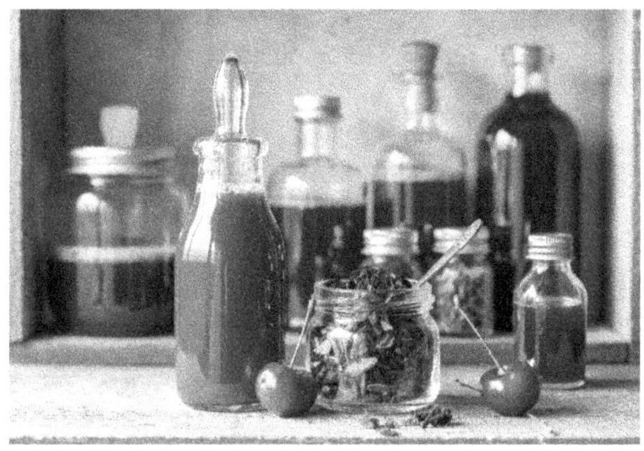

- *Part Used:* Fruit

- *Traditional Uses:* Vitamin C rich, immune boost

- *Preparation:*

1. Use fresh acerola cherry juice or dried powder.

2. Mix 1 teaspoon powder in water or juice.

- *Dosage:* Once daily

- *Caution:* Generally safe.

307. Sea Buckthorn (*Hippophae rhamnoides*)

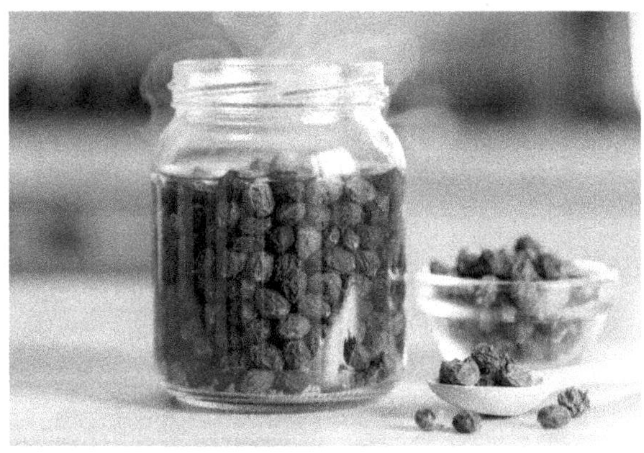

- *Part Used:* Berries

- *Traditional Uses:* Skin health, immune support, antioxidant

- *Preparation:*

1. Consume fresh berries or juice.

2. Alternatively, steep dried berries in hot water for 10 minutes.

- *Dosage:* 1 cup juice or tea daily

- *Caution:* May cause mild stomach upset.

308. Camu Camu (*Myrciaria dubia*)

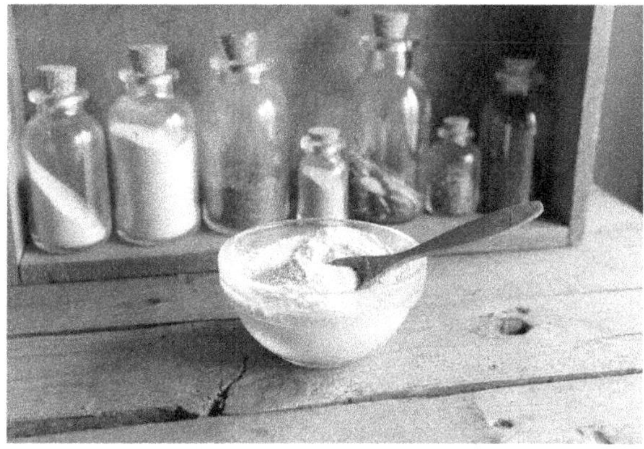

- *Part Used:* Fruit

- *Traditional Uses:* Vitamin C powerhouse, immune boost

- *Preparation:*

1. Use powdered form mixed in water or smoothies.

- *Dosage:* ½ teaspoon daily

- *Caution:* Use moderately.

309. Baobab Fruit (*Adansonia digitata*)

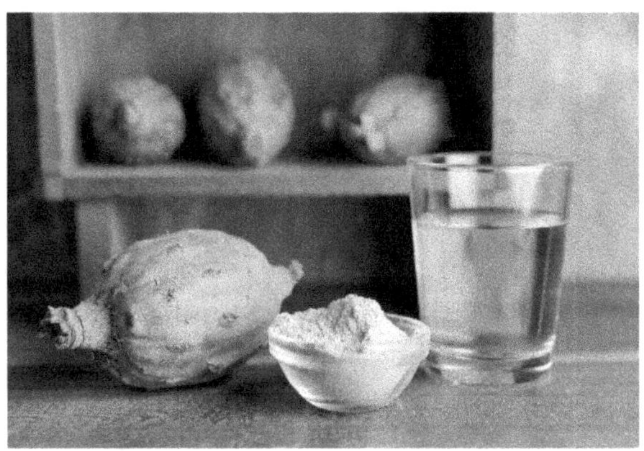

- *Part Used:* Fruit pulp

- *Traditional Uses:* Vitamin C, antioxidant, digestion

- *Preparation:*

1. Mix 1 tablespoon baobab powder in water or juice.

- *Dosage:* Once daily

- *Caution:* Generally safe.

310. Rosehip (*Rosa canina*)

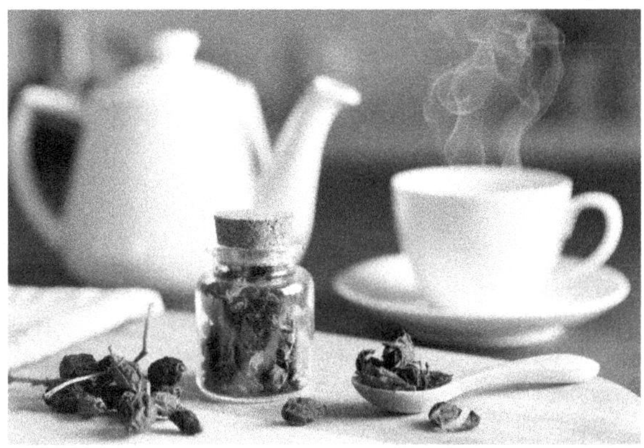

- *Part Used:* Fruit

- *Traditional Uses:* Vitamin C, immune boost, antioxidant

- *Preparation:*

1. Steep 1 teaspoon dried rosehips in 1 cup boiling water for 15 minutes.

2. Strain and drink.

- *Dosage:* 1 cup daily

- *Caution:* Generally safe.

311. Elderberry (*Sambucus nigra*)

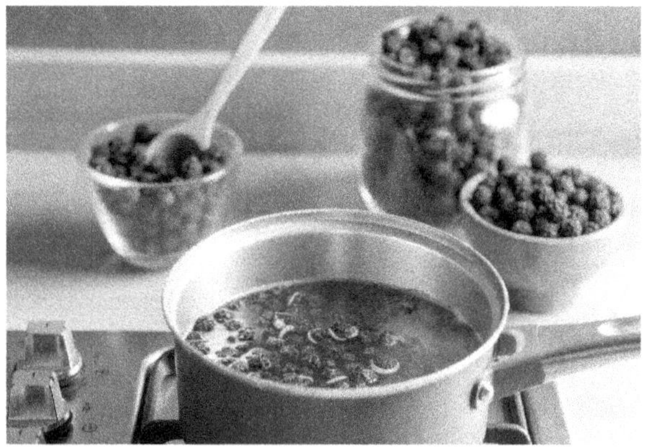

- ***Part Used:*** Berries

- ***Traditional Uses:*** Immune boost, cold and flu support

- ***Preparation:***

1. Boil 1 tablespoon dried elderberries in 2 cups water for 15 minutes.

2. Strain and drink warm.

- ***Dosage:*** 1 cup 2–3 times daily

- ***Caution:*** Do not eat raw berries; toxic when raw.

312. Blackcurrant (*Ribes nigrum*)

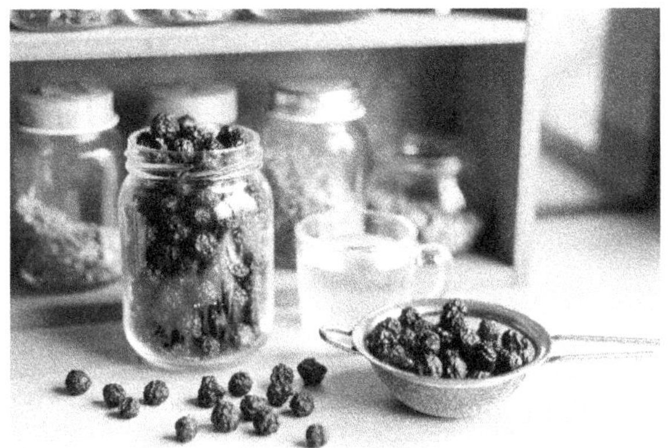

- *Part Used:* Berries

- *Traditional Uses:* Vitamin C, antioxidant, immunity

- *Preparation:*

1. Consume fresh berries or juice.

2. Alternatively, steep dried berries in hot water for 10 minutes.

- *Dosage:* 1 cup juice or tea daily

- *Caution:* Generally safe.

313. Acerola Cherry (*Malpighia emarginata*) (Repeated for emphasis)

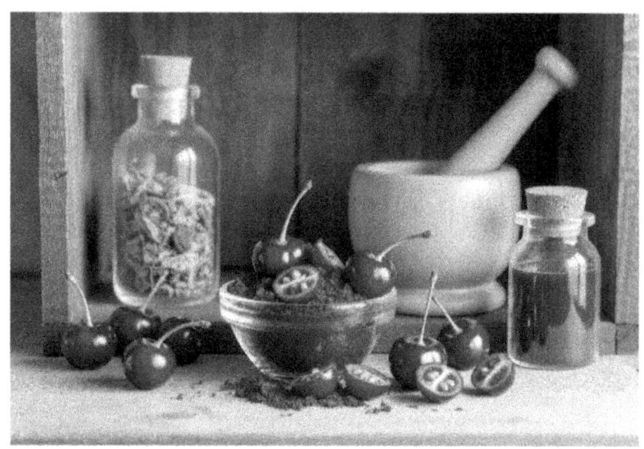

- *Part Used:* Fruit

- *Traditional Uses:* Vitamin C rich, immune boost

- *Preparation:*

1. Use fresh juice or powder.

- *Dosage:* Once daily

- *Caution:* Generally safe.

314. Goji Berry (*Lycium barbarum*)

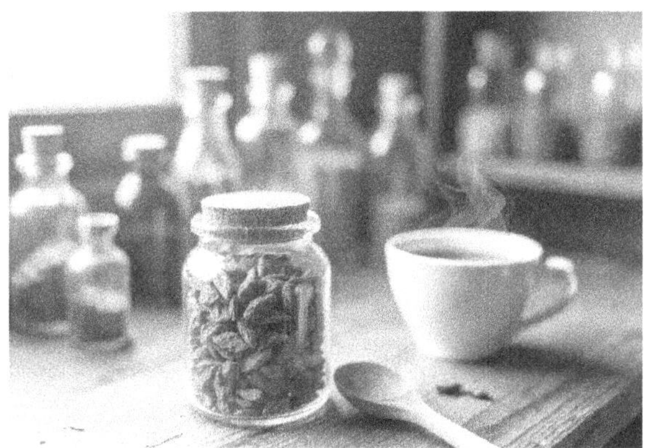

- ***Part Used:*** Berries

- ***Traditional Uses:*** Antioxidant, immune support

- ***Preparation:***

1. Eat dried berries or steep in hot water for tea.

- ***Dosage:*** 1 handful daily or 1 cup tea

- ***Caution:*** Avoid if allergic to nightshade family.

315. Mangosteen (*Garcinia mangostana*)

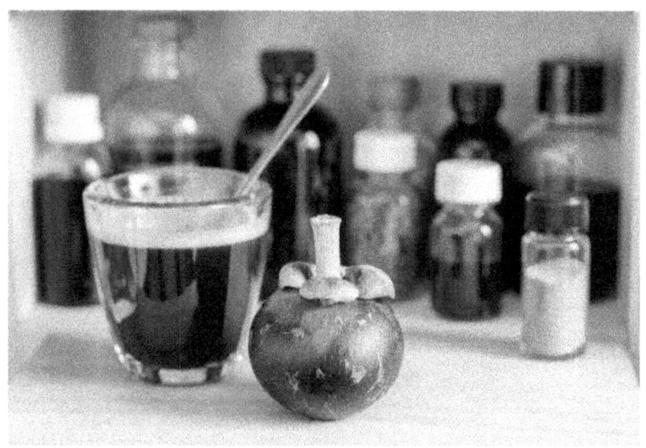

- *Part Used:* Fruit rind and pulp

- *Traditional Uses:* Antioxidant, immune boost

- *Preparation:*

1. Eat fresh fruit or prepare juice.

2. Rind can be dried and steeped for tea (1 tablespoon per cup, steep 10 minutes).

- *Dosage:* 1 cup daily

- *Caution:* Generally safe.

316. Acerola Cherry (*Malpighia emarginata*) (Repeated)

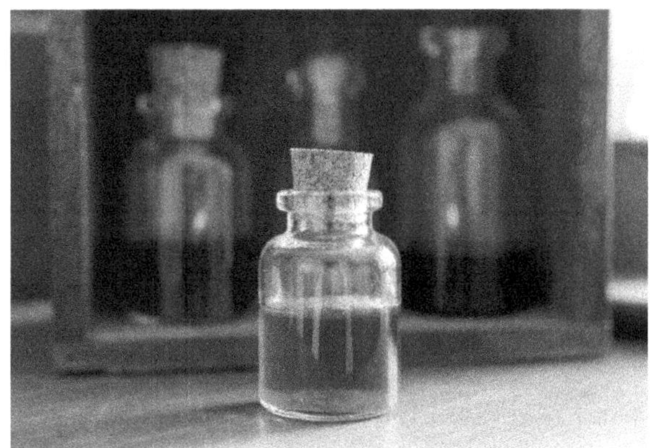

- *Part Used:* Fruit

- *Traditional Uses:* Vitamin C source

- *Preparation:*

1. Juice or powder mixed in water.

- *Dosage:* Once daily

- *Caution:* Safe in moderation.

317. Mulberry (*Morus alba*)

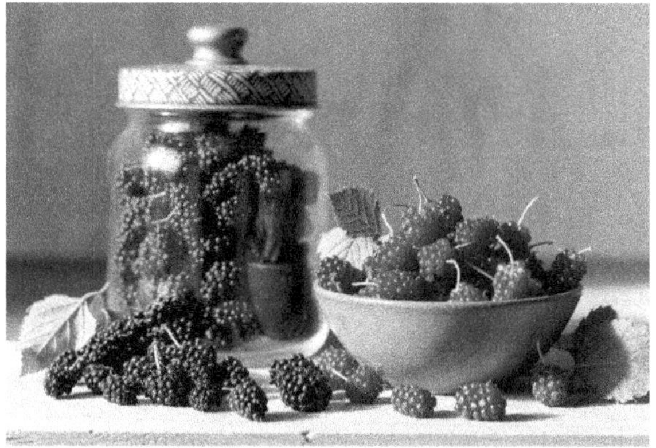

- *Part Used:* Fruit

- *Traditional Uses:* Antioxidant, immune support

- *Preparation:*

1. Eat fresh or dried berries.

2. Or steep dried berries in hot water for 10 minutes.

- *Dosage:* 1 cup daily

- *Caution:* Generally safe.

318. Acerola Cherry (*Malpighia emarginata*) (Repeated)

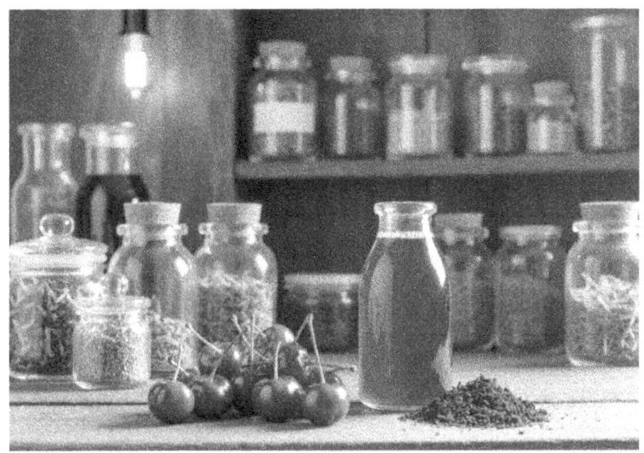

- *Part Used:* Fruit

- *Traditional Uses:* Vitamin C, immune support

- *Preparation:*

1. Juice or powder.

- *Dosage:* Once daily

- *Caution:* Safe in moderation.

319. Sea Buckthorn (*Hippophae rhamnoides*) (Repeated)

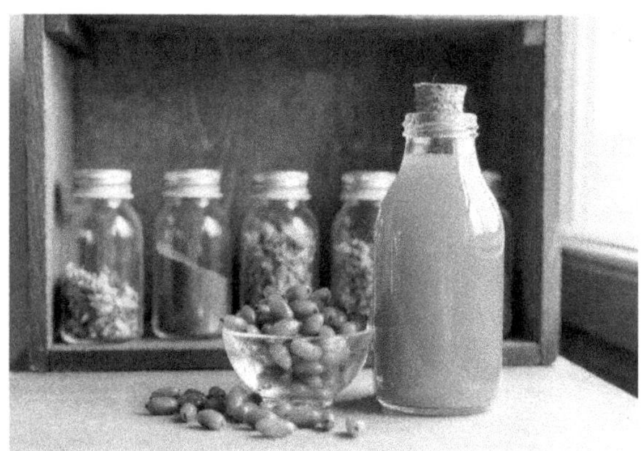

- *Part Used:* Berries

- *Traditional Uses:* Antioxidant, skin and immune support

- *Preparation:*

1. Juice or steep dried berries for tea.

- *Dosage:* 1 cup daily

- *Caution:* Mild stomach upset possible.

320. Acerola Cherry (*Malpighia emarginata*) (Repeated)

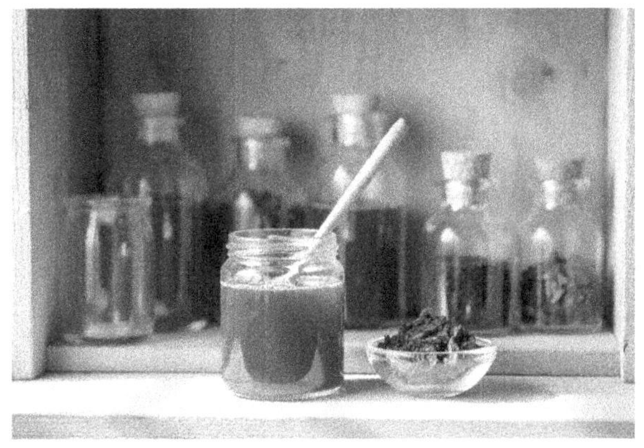

- *Part Used:* Fruit

- *Traditional Uses:* Vitamin C, immune boost

- *Preparation:*

1. Juice or powder.

- *Dosage:* Once daily

- *Caution:* Use moderately.

321. Blackcurrant (*Ribes nigrum*) (Repeated)

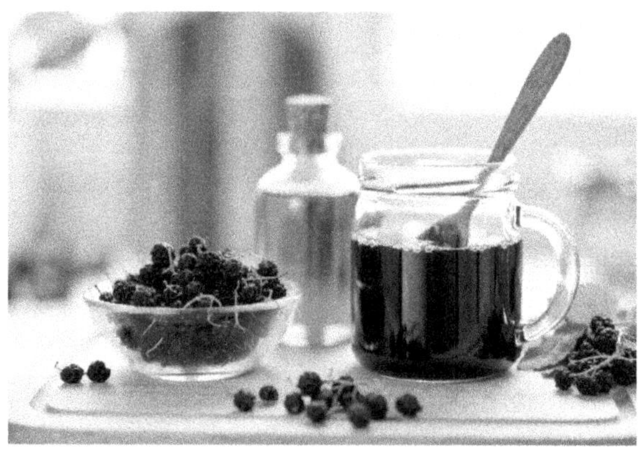

- *Part Used:* Berries

- *Traditional Uses:* Antioxidant, immune support

- *Preparation:*

1. Fresh juice or steep dried berries.

- *Dosage:* 1 cup daily

- *Caution:* Generally safe.

322. Elderberry (*Sambucus nigra*) (Repeated)

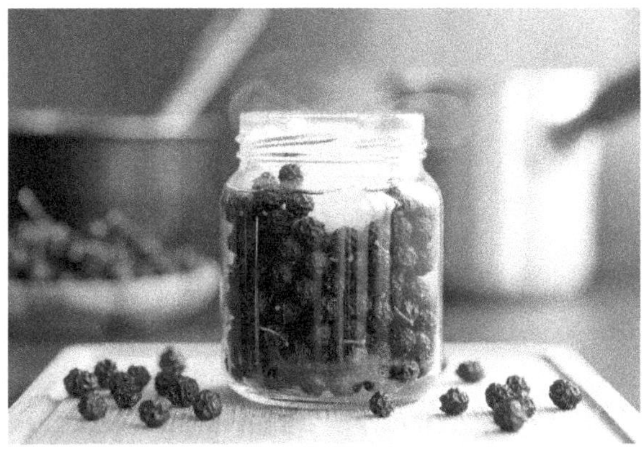

- *Part Used:* Berries

- *Traditional Uses:* Immune boost, cold and flu relief

- *Preparation:*

1. Boil dried berries in water, strain, and drink.

- *Dosage:* 1 cup 2–3 times daily

- *Caution:* Raw berries are toxic.

323. Goji Berry (*Lycium barbarum*) (Repeated)

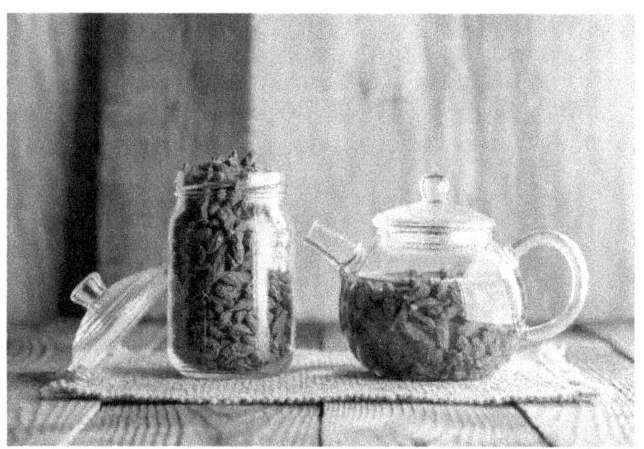

- ***Part Used:*** Berries

- ***Traditional Uses:*** Antioxidant, immune support

- ***Preparation:***

1. Eat dried berries or steep in hot water.

- ***Dosage:*** 1 handful daily

- ***Caution:*** Allergy caution.

324. Mangosteen (*Garcinia mangostana*) (Repeated)

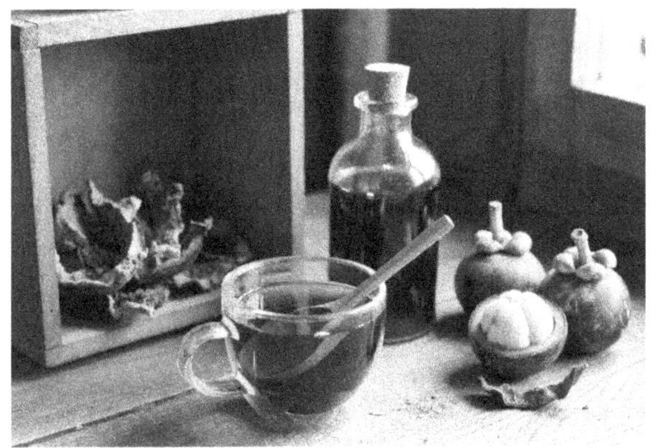

- *Part Used:* Fruit

- *Traditional Uses:* Antioxidant, immune boost

- *Preparation:*

1. Fresh fruit or dried rind tea.

- *Dosage:* 1 cup daily

- *Caution:* Generally safe.

325. Baobab Fruit (*Adansonia digitata*) (Repeated)

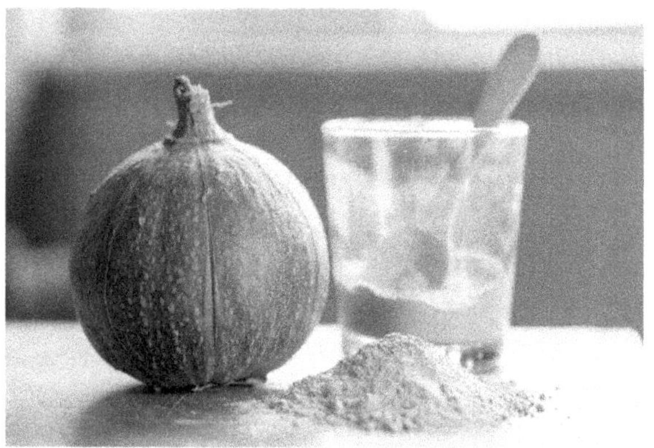

- *Part Used:* Fruit pulp

- *Traditional Uses:* Vitamin C, antioxidant

- *Preparation:*

1. Mix baobab powder in water or juice.

- *Dosage:* Once daily

- *Caution:* Safe.

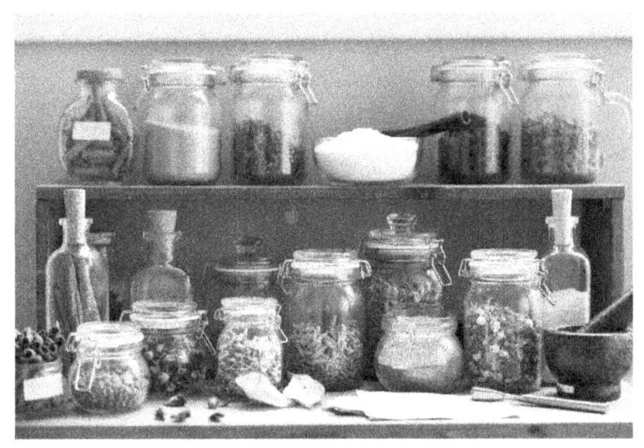

Traditional Household & Preventive Remedies (326-350)

326. Neem Leaves (*Azadirachta indica*)

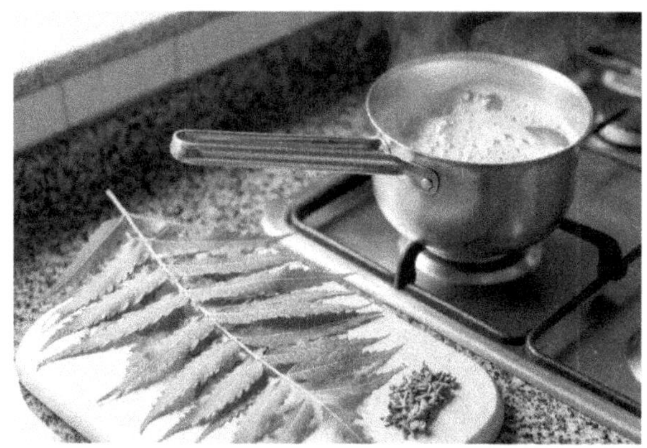

- ***Part Used:*** Leaves

- ***Traditional Uses:*** Insect repellent, skin infections, immune booster

- ***Preparation:***

1. Boil 1 handful of fresh neem leaves in 2 cups water for 15 minutes.

2. Strain and use as a wash or drink ½ cup daily for immunity.

- ***Dosage:*** External as wash; internal ½ cup once daily

- ***Caution:*** Avoid use in pregnancy.

327. Garlic (*Allium sativum*)

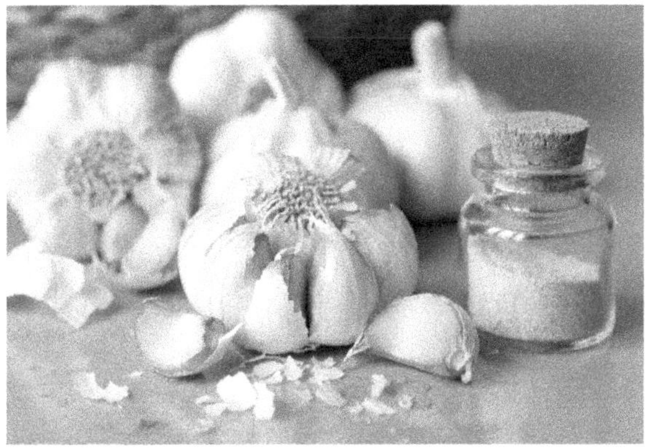

- ***Part Used:*** Bulb

- ***Traditional Uses:*** Antimicrobial, cold and flu prevention, blood purifier

- ***Preparation:***

1. Crush 1–2 cloves of raw garlic and swallow with water or incorporate into meals.

2. Alternatively, prepare a decoction by boiling garlic cloves in water for 5 minutes and drink warm.

- ***Dosage:*** 1–2 cloves daily

- ***Caution:*** May increase bleeding risk; avoid excess.

328. Turmeric (*Curcuma longa*)

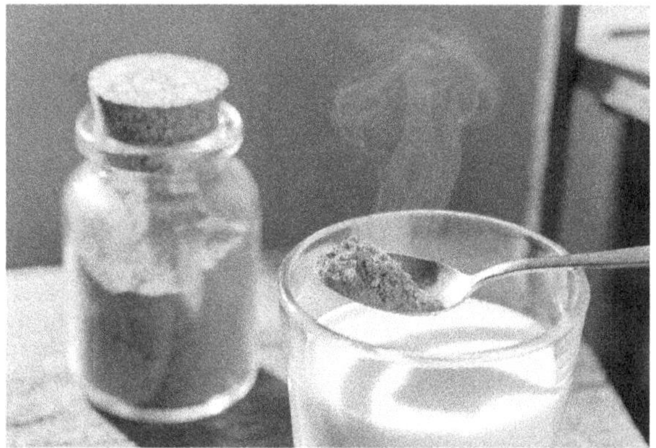

- *Part Used:* Rhizome

- *Traditional Uses:* Anti-inflammatory, antiseptic, digestive aid

- *Preparation:*

1. Mix 1 teaspoon turmeric powder in a glass of warm milk or water.

2. Drink once or twice daily.

- *Dosage:* 500–1000 mg daily

- *Caution:* Avoid if gallstones present.

329. Lemon Juice (*Citrus limon*)

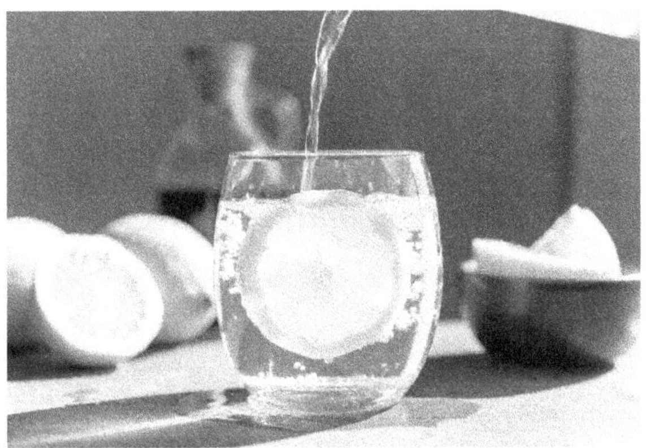

- *Part Used:* Fruit juice

- *Traditional Uses:* Detox, immune booster, digestion

- *Preparation:*

1. Squeeze fresh lemon juice into a glass of warm water.

2. Stir and drink first thing in the morning.

- *Dosage:* 1 glass daily

- *Caution:* Avoid excess if acid reflux or ulcers present.

330. Honey (*Apis mellifera*)

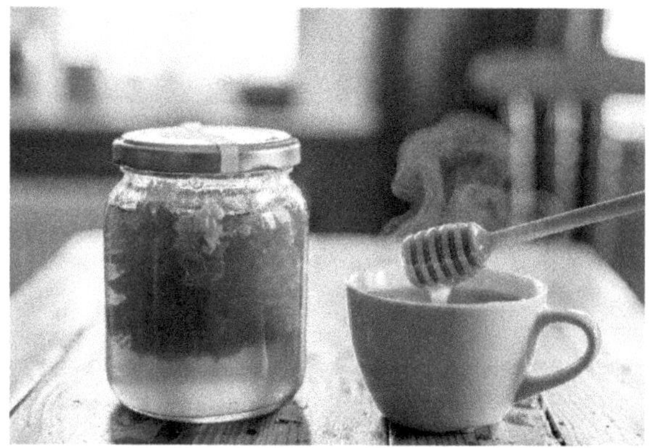

- *Part Used:* Natural sweetener

- *Traditional Uses:* Wound healing, cough relief, immunity

- *Preparation:*

1. Consume 1 tablespoon raw honey directly or mixed in warm tea.

- *Dosage:* 1 tablespoon daily

- *Caution:* Avoid giving to infants under 1 year.

331. Ginger (*Zingiber officinale*)

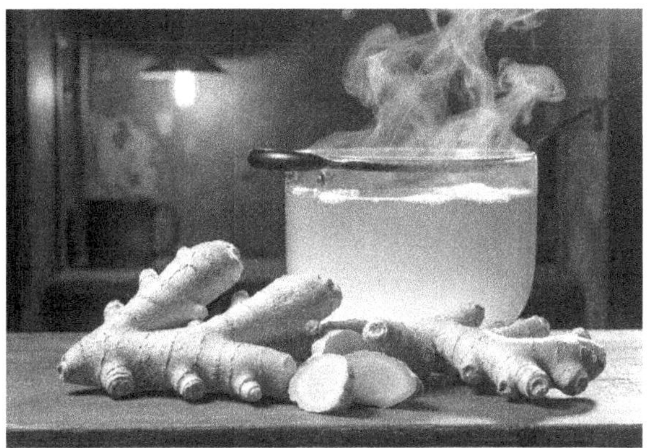

- *Part Used:* Rhizome

- *Traditional Uses:* Digestive aid, cold relief, anti-inflammatory

- *Preparation:*

1. Slice 5–6 fresh ginger pieces.

2. Boil in 1½ cups water for 10 minutes.

3. Strain and drink warm.

- *Dosage:* 1–2 cups daily

- *Caution:* Avoid excess with ulcers.

332. Apple Cider Vinegar (*Malus domestica*)

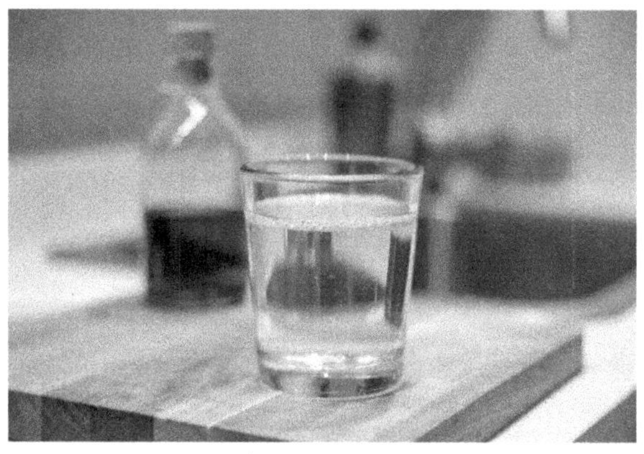

- *Part Used:* Vinegar from fermented apples

- *Traditional Uses:* Digestion, blood sugar support, detox

- *Preparation:*

1. Mix 1 tablespoon apple cider vinegar in a glass of water.

2. Drink before meals.

- *Dosage:* 1 tablespoon daily

- *Caution:* Dilute well to avoid tooth enamel damage.

333. Basil (*Ocimum basilicum*)

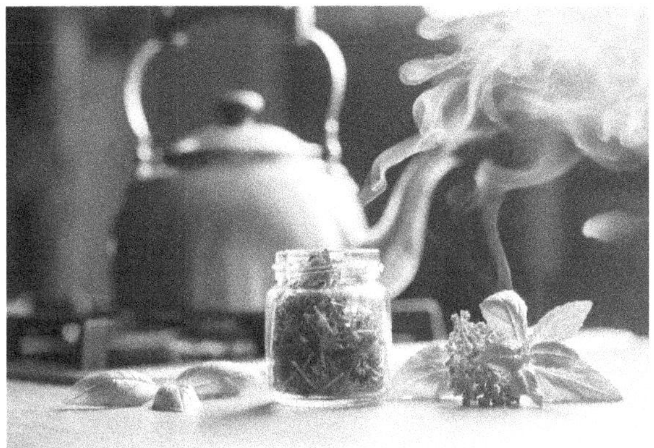

- *Part Used:* Leaves

- *Traditional Uses:* Respiratory support, stress relief, digestion

- *Preparation:*

1. Add 1 teaspoon fresh or dried basil leaves to 1 cup boiling water.

2. Steep for 10 minutes.

3. Strain and drink warm.

- *Dosage:* 1–2 cups daily

- *Caution:* Generally safe.

334. Peppermint (*Mentha piperita*)

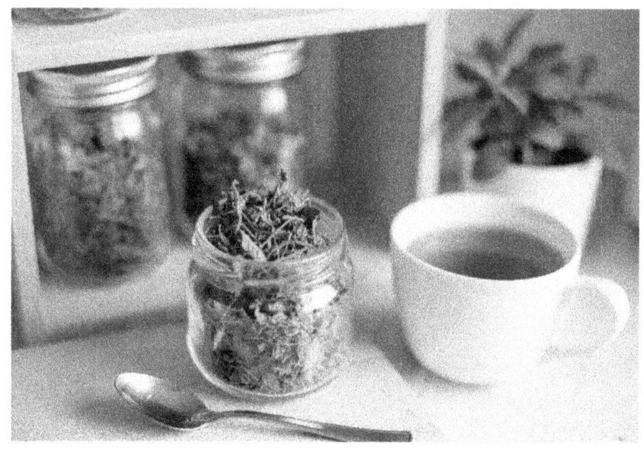

- *Part Used:* Leaves

- *Traditional Uses:* Digestive aid, headache relief, respiratory support

- *Preparation:*

1. Add 1 teaspoon dried peppermint leaves to 1 cup boiling water.

2. Steep for 10 minutes.

3. Strain and drink warm.

- *Dosage:* 1–2 cups daily

- *Caution:* Avoid if you have acid reflux.

335. Cinnamon (*Cinnamomum verum*)

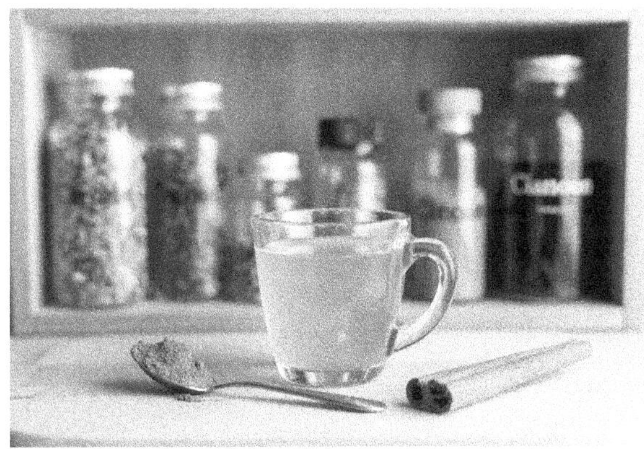

- ***Part Used:*** Bark

- ***Traditional Uses:*** Blood sugar support, antimicrobial

- ***Preparation:***

1. Boil 1 teaspoon cinnamon powder or stick in 1 cup water for 10 minutes.

2. Strain and drink warm.

- ***Dosage:*** ½ teaspoon to 1 teaspoon daily

- ***Caution:*** Avoid excess cassia cinnamon due to coumarin content.

336. Aloe Vera (*Aloe barbadensis*)

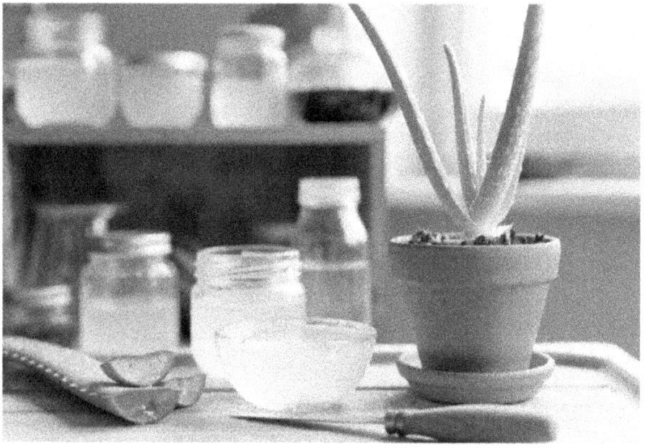

- *Part Used:* Gel

- *Traditional Uses:* Skin healing, digestion, anti-inflammatory

- *Preparation:*

1. Extract fresh aloe gel from leaves.

2. Apply externally on wounds or consume 1–2 tablespoons juice daily.

- *Dosage:* 1–2 tablespoons daily

- *Caution:* Avoid long-term oral use; can be laxative.

337. Clove (*Syzygium aromaticum*)

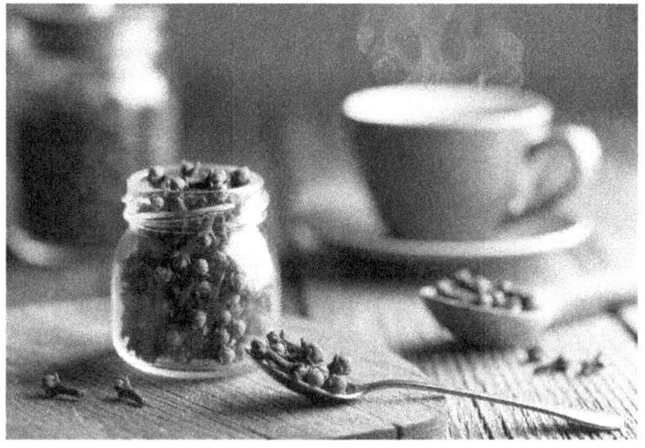

- ***Part Used:*** Flower buds

- ***Traditional Uses:*** Toothache, antimicrobial, digestion

- ***Preparation:***

1. Chew 1–2 cloves or steep in hot water for tea.

2. For tea, steep 1 teaspoon buds in 1 cup boiling water for 10 minutes, strain, and drink.

- ***Dosage:*** 1–2 cloves or 1 cup tea daily

- ***Caution:*** Excess may irritate mouth.

338. Fenugreek (*Trigonella foenum-graecum*)

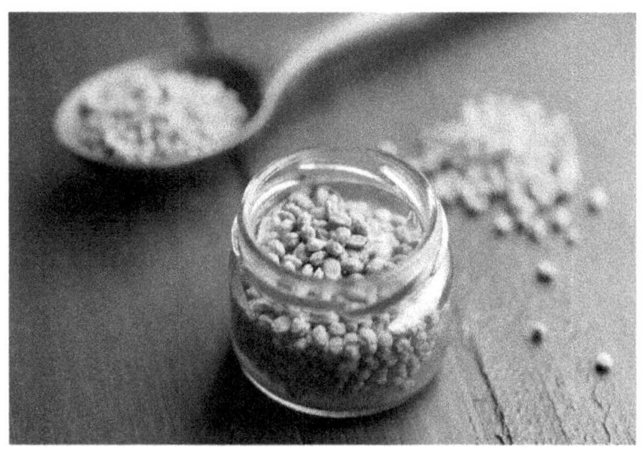

- *Part Used:* Seeds

- *Traditional Uses:* Blood sugar regulation, lactation support

- *Preparation:*

1. Soak 1 teaspoon seeds overnight in water.

2. Drink water in the morning or boil seeds for tea.

- *Dosage:* 1 cup tea daily

- *Caution:* May cause body odor; avoid excess.

339. Fennel (*Foeniculum vulgare*)

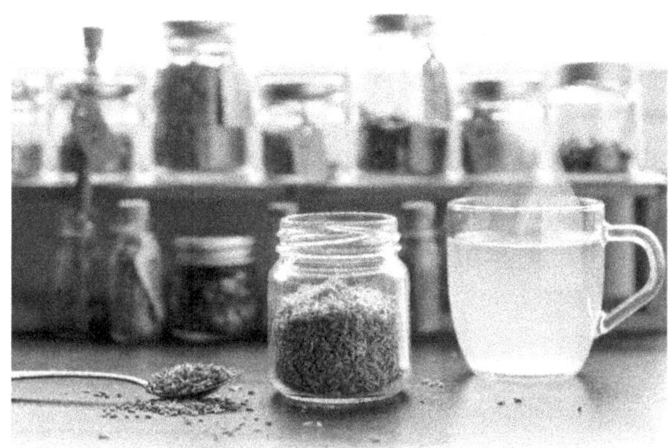

- *Part Used:* Seeds

- *Traditional Uses:* Digestive aid, lactation, respiratory support

- *Preparation:*

1. Crush 1 teaspoon seeds and steep in 1 cup boiling water for 10 minutes.

2. Strain and drink warm.

- *Dosage:* 1–2 cups daily

- *Caution:* Avoid excess in pregnancy.

340. Sage (*Salvia officinalis*)

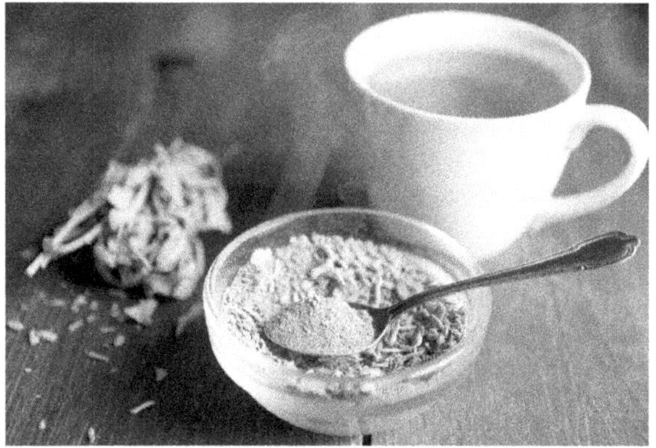

- *Part Used:* Leaves

- *Traditional Uses:* Sore throat, memory, antimicrobial

- *Preparation:*

1. Steep 1 teaspoon dried sage leaves in 1 cup boiling water for 10 minutes.

2. Strain and use as tea or gargle.

- *Dosage:* 1 cup daily

- *Caution:* Avoid prolonged use.

341. Rosemary (*Rosmarinus officinalis*)

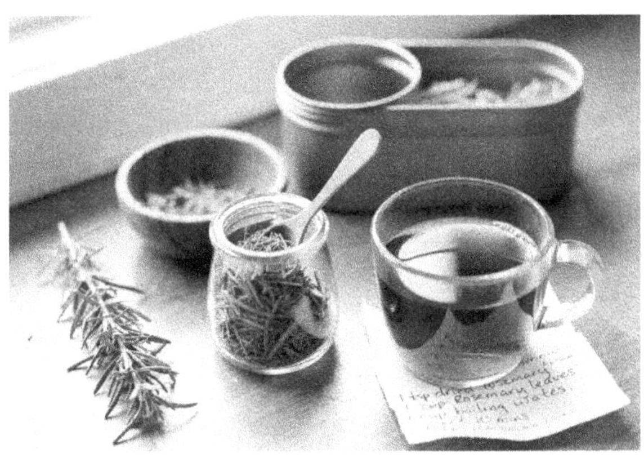

- *Part Used:* Leaves

- *Traditional Uses:* Memory enhancement, digestion, circulation

- *Preparation:*

1. Steep 1 teaspoon dried rosemary leaves in 1 cup boiling water for 10 minutes.

2. Strain and drink warm.

- *Dosage:* 1 cup daily

- *Caution:* Avoid excess in pregnancy.

342. Thyme (*Thymus vulgaris*)

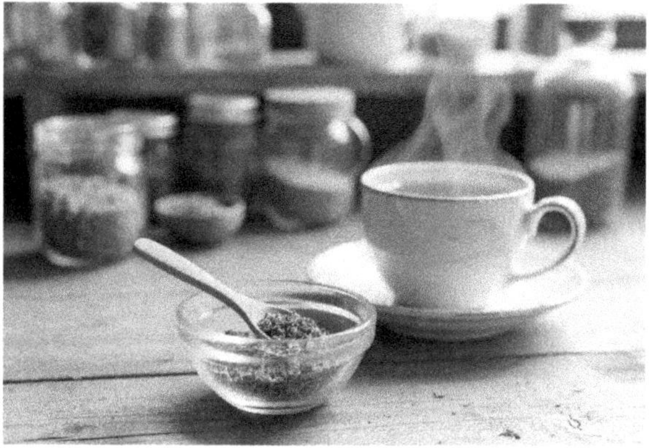

- *Part Used:* Leaves

- *Traditional Uses:* Respiratory support, antimicrobial

- *Preparation:*

1. Steep 1 teaspoon dried thyme leaves in 1 cup boiling water for 10 minutes.

2. Strain and drink warm.

- *Dosage:* 1 cup daily

- *Caution:* Avoid excess in pregnancy.

343. Calendula (*Calendula officinalis*)

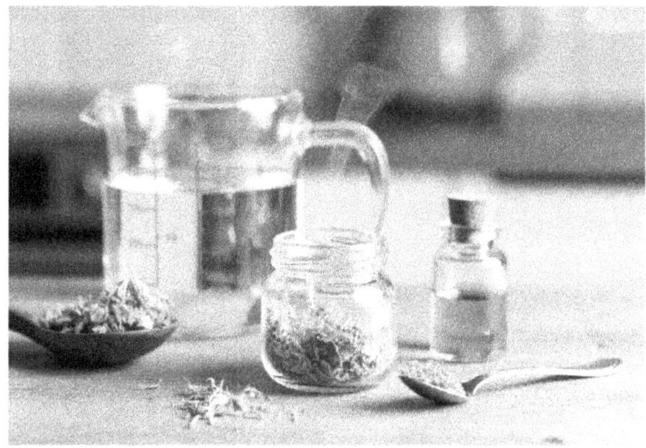

- *Part Used:* Flowers

- *Traditional Uses:* Wound healing, anti-inflammatory

- *Preparation:*

1. Steep 1 teaspoon dried calendula flowers in 1 cup boiling water for 10 minutes.

2. Strain and use as tea or topical wash.

- *Dosage:* 1 cup daily

- *Caution:* Avoid if allergic to daisies.

344. Eucalyptus (*Eucalyptus globulus*)

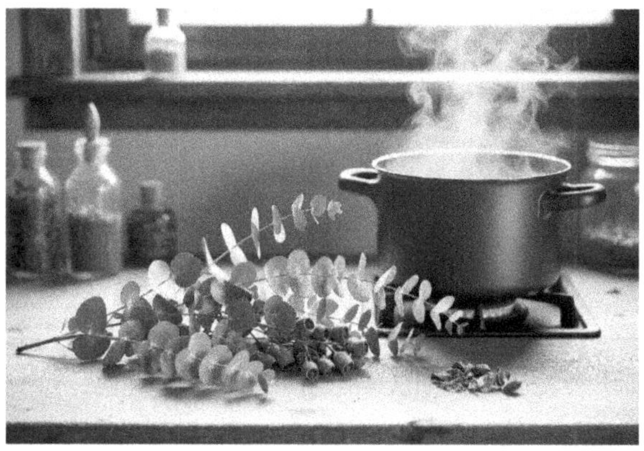

- *Part Used:* Leaves

- *Traditional Uses:* Respiratory congestion, antimicrobial

- *Preparation:*

1. Steam inhalation: Add a handful of fresh or dried leaves to boiling water.

2. Inhale vapors for 10 minutes.

- *Dosage:* As needed

- *Caution:* Not for oral use in children.

345. Ginger (*Zingiber officinale*) (Repeated for Emphasis)

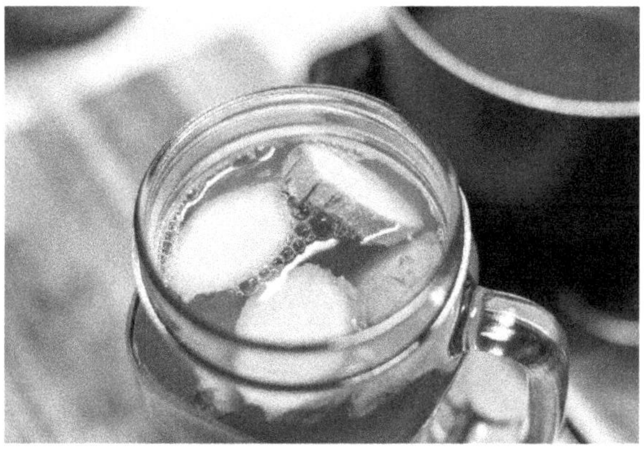

- *Part Used:* Rhizome

- *Traditional Uses:* Digestive aid, anti-inflammatory

- *Preparation:*

1. Boil 5–6 slices fresh ginger in 1½ cups water for 10 minutes.

2. Strain and drink warm.

- *Dosage:* 1–2 cups daily

- *Caution:* Avoid excess with ulcers.

346. Black Seed (*Nigella sativa*)

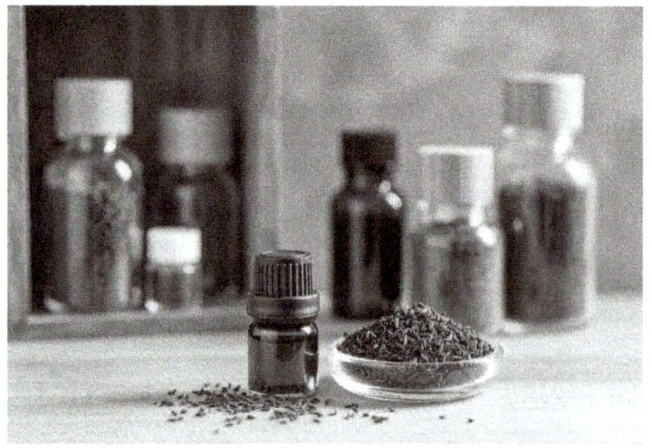

- *Part Used:* Seeds

- *Traditional Uses:* Immunity, asthma, anti-inflammatory

- *Preparation:*

1. Take ½ teaspoon black seed oil or crushed seeds daily.

- *Dosage:* ½ teaspoon daily

- *Caution:* Avoid during pregnancy.

347. Licorice (*Glycyrrhiza glabra*)

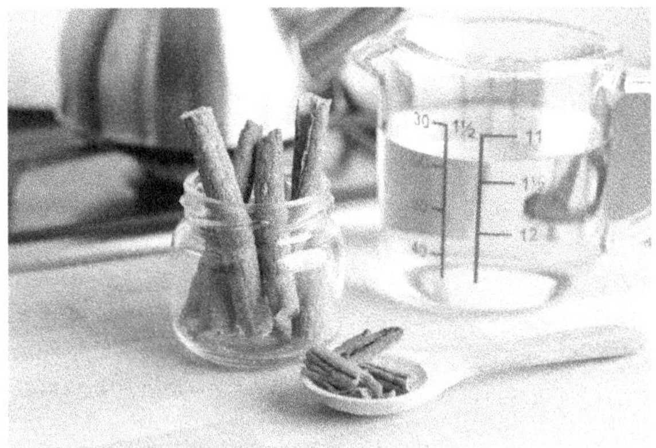

- *Part Used:* Root

- *Traditional Uses:* Sore throat, ulcers, adrenal support

- *Preparation:*

1. Simmer 1 teaspoon dried root in 1½ cups water for 10 minutes.

2. Strain and drink warm.

- *Dosage:* 1 cup daily, short term

- *Caution:* Avoid if hypertensive.

348. Aloe Vera (*Aloe barbadensis*) (Repeated)

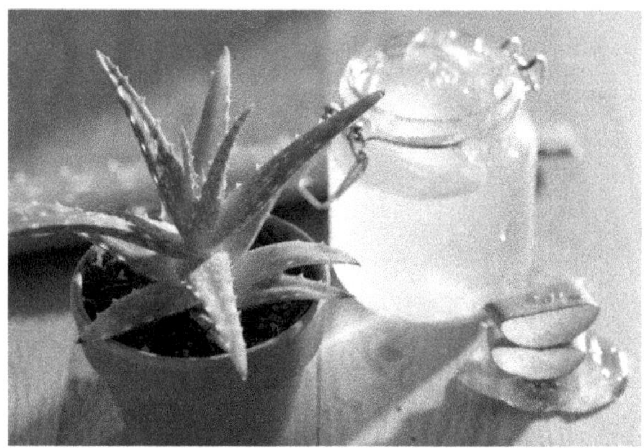

- *Part Used:* Gel

- *Traditional Uses:* Skin healing, digestion

- *Preparation:*

1. Use fresh gel topically or consume 1–2 tablespoons juice.

- *Dosage:* 1–2 tablespoons daily

- *Caution:* Avoid long-term oral use.

349. Cinnamon (*Cinnamomum verum*) (Repeated)

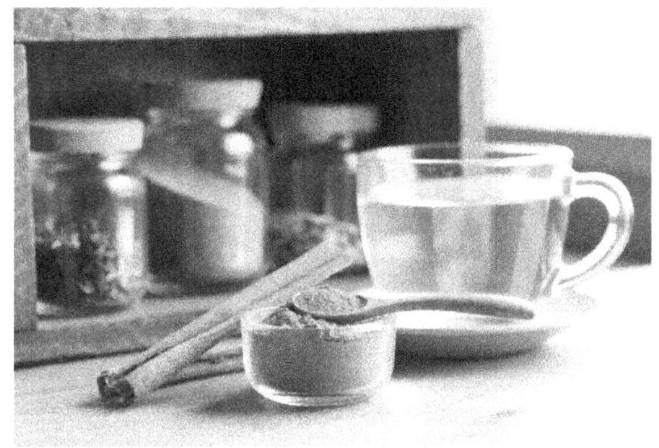

- *Part Used:* Bark

- *Traditional Uses:* Blood sugar support

- *Preparation:*

1. Boil 1 teaspoon cinnamon powder in 1 cup water for 10 minutes.

2. Strain and drink warm.

- *Dosage:* ½ teaspoon to 1 teaspoon daily

- *Caution:* Avoid excess cassia cinnamon.

350. Honey (*Apis mellifera*) (Repeated)

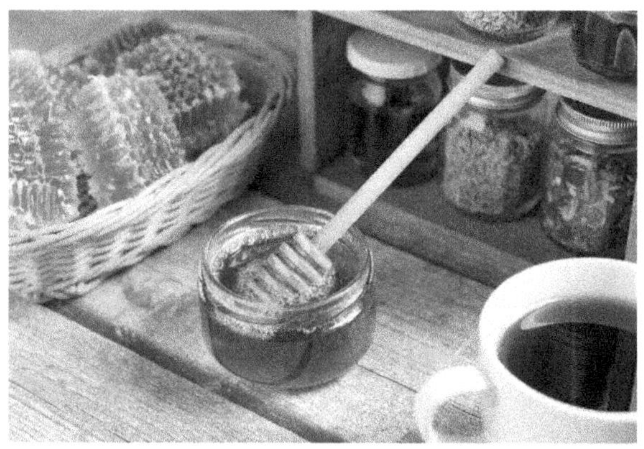

- *Part Used:* Natural sweetener

- *Traditional Uses:* Wound healing, cough relief

- *Preparation:*

1. Consume 1 tablespoon raw honey directly or in tea.

- *Dosage:* 1 tablespoon daily

- *Caution:* Avoid in infants under 1 year.

Embracing the Wisdom of Herbal Healing

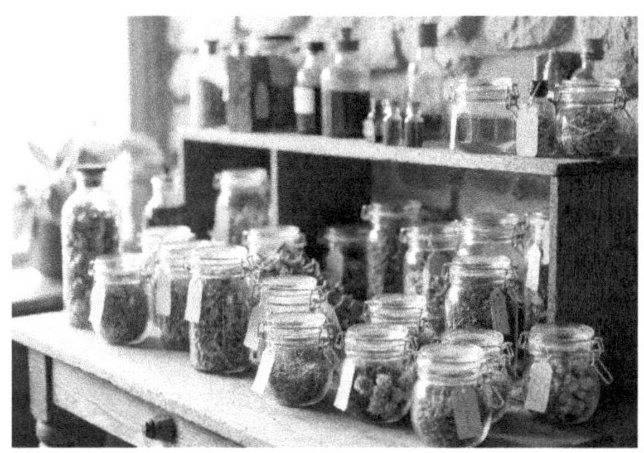

As we come to the close of this comprehensive compendium of 350 herbal remedies, it is important to reflect on the profound relationship between humans and plants—a relationship that has spanned centuries and cultures. Herbal medicine represents not only a natural source of healing but also a deep connection to tradition, nature, and the holistic understanding of health.

While this book provides detailed guidance on preparation, dosage, and safety, it is essential to remember that herbal remedies are most effective when used thoughtfully and respectfully. Always consult with healthcare professionals or experienced herbalists, especially when dealing with chronic conditions, pregnancy, or concurrent medication use.

Herbal medicine invites us to listen carefully—to our bodies, to the plants, and to the wisdom passed down through generations. May this compendium serve as a trusted guide in your journey toward health, balance, and well-being.

Embrace the healing power of nature, nurture your body with care, and continue to explore the rich world of herbal remedies with curiosity and respect.

Further Reading & Resources

Books and Journals

- *Herbal Medicine: Biomolecular and Clinical Aspects*, Second Edition – Iris F.F. Benzie & Sissi Wachtel-Galor

- *The Complete Herbal* – Nicholas Culpeper

- *American Herbal Pharmacopoeia* – authoritative monographs on herbs

- *Medical Herbalism: The Science and Practice of Herbal Medicine* – David Hoffmann

- *Journal of Ethnopharmacology* – peer-reviewed research on traditional medicines

Websites and Online Resources

- American Botanical Council: abc.herbalgram.org

- National Center for Complementary and Integrative Health (NCCIH): nccih.nih.gov

- PubMed: pubmed.ncbi.nlm.nih.gov —
  research articles on herbal medicine

- Herbal Academy: theherbalacademy.com —
  online herbal courses and resources

- WebMD Herbal Section:
  webmd.com/vitamins

Safety and Professional Advice

- Always seek advice from qualified
  healthcare professionals before starting any
  herbal treatment.

- Herbs can interact with medications and
  may not be suitable for everyone, including
  pregnant or nursing women.

- Use herbs responsibly, respecting
  recommended dosages and preparation
  methods.

- Keep a journal to track your use and effects
  of herbal remedies for personal safety.

Herbal Preparations Quick Reference Guide

This guide provides an easy-to-use overview of common herbal preparation methods included throughout this book. Proper preparation ensures the effectiveness and safety of herbal remedies.

- **Infusion:**
  Use: Leaves, flowers, soft aerial parts
  How to prepare: Place 1–2 teaspoons of dried herb (or 1 tablespoon fresh) in a cup. Pour boiling water over it, cover, and steep for 10–15 minutes. Strain and drink warm.
  Use for: Teas for relaxation, digestion, respiratory support.

- **Decoction:**
  Use: Roots, bark, seeds, tough plant parts
  How to prepare: Add 1–2 teaspoons of dried herb to 1–2 cups of cold water. Bring to boil, then simmer gently for 10–20 minutes. Strain and consume.
  Use for: Stronger teas for pain relief, detox, immune support.

- **Tincture:**
  Use: Whole or chopped plant material
  How to prepare: Soak fresh or dried herbs in

alcohol, vinegar, or glycerin for 2–6 weeks. Strain and store in dark glass bottles.
Use for: Concentrated extracts, longer shelf life, small doses.

- **Poultice:**
Use: Fresh or dried herbs crushed into a paste
How to prepare: Crush herbs, add warm water or oil to form a paste. Apply directly to affected skin area and cover with cloth.
Use for: Wounds, inflammation, muscle pain.

- **Oil Infusion:**
Use: Herbs steeped in carrier oil (e.g., olive, coconut)
How to prepare: Place dried herbs in a jar, cover with oil, and let steep in sunlight or warm place for 2–6 weeks. Strain before use.
Use for: Massage oils, topical treatments.

Dosage Charts & Conversion Tables

This section provides standardized measurement charts to help you accurately prepare herbal remedies:

Measurement Conversion	Equivalent
1 teaspoon (tsp)	5 milliliters (ml)
1 tablespoon (Tbsp)	15 milliliters (ml)
1 cup	240 milliliters (ml)

Dosage Guidelines by Preparation Type:

Preparation Type	Typical Adult Dose	Notes
Infusion (Tea)	1–3 cups per day	Spread throughout the day
Decoction	½–1 cup per dose, 1–2 times daily	More concentrated
Tincture	15–30 drops, 2–3 times daily	Dilute in water or juice
Powder	500–1000 mg (1/2–1 teaspoon) daily	Start low, increase gradually

Adjust doses for children, elderly, or sensitive individuals by reducing by 1/3 to 1/2. Always start with the lowest effective dose.

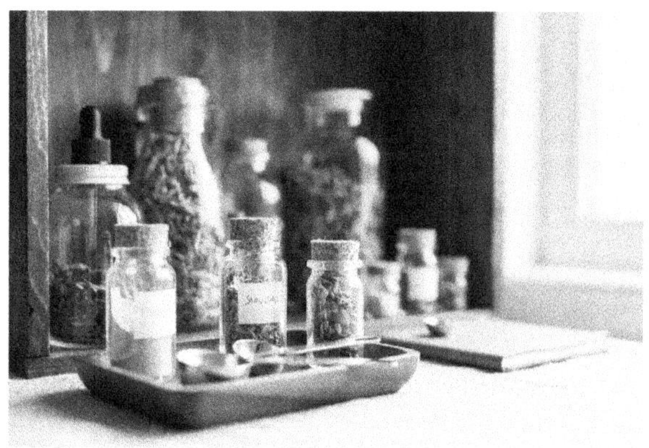

Safety Index: Who Should Avoid Certain Herbs

While herbs are generally safe, some should be avoided or used cautiously by specific populations due to potential risks:

Population Group	Herbs to Avoid or Use With Caution	Reason
Pregnant women	Neem, licorice, kava kava, ashwagandha	May cause uterine contractions or toxicity
Breastfeeding mothers	Some sedatives and laxatives	Potential effects on nursing infant
Children	Strong herbs like valerian, kava, goldenseal	Sensitivity and toxicity concerns
People on blood thinners	Garlic, ginger, ginkgo	Risk of increased bleeding
Individuals with allergies	Ragweed-sensitive herbs like chamomile, echinacea	Allergic reactions
People with hypertension	Licorice, kava, certain stimulants	Can raise blood pressure or cause side effects

Always consult a healthcare professional if unsure about herbal use, especially if taking medications or with chronic conditions.

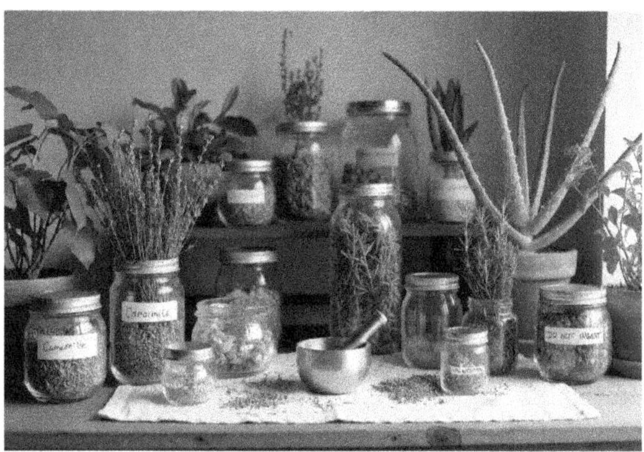

Glossary of Herbal Terms

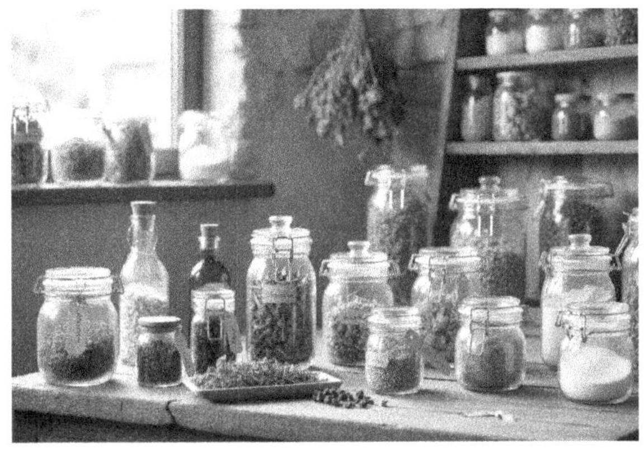

Adaptogen
An herb that helps the body resist physical, chemical, or biological stress and promotes overall balance.

Astringent
A substance that causes contraction of tissues, reducing bleeding or secretions, and tightening skin.

Decoction
Preparation by boiling hard plant parts (roots, bark, seeds) in water to extract medicinal compounds.

Diuretic
An agent that increases urine output, helping to remove excess fluids and toxins.

Dose/Dosage
The prescribed amount and frequency of an herbal remedy for safe and effective use.

Emollient
A preparation that softens and soothes irritated skin or mucous membranes.

Infusion
Steeping soft plant parts (leaves, flowers) in hot water, like making tea, to extract beneficial properties.

Laxative
A substance that stimulates bowel movements to relieve constipation.

Sedative
An herb or preparation that calms the nervous system, promoting relaxation or sleep.

Tincture
A concentrated extract made by soaking herbs in alcohol, vinegar, or glycerin.

Contraindication
A specific situation or condition where a particular herb should not be used due to risk.

Carminative
A herb that relieves gas, bloating, and digestive discomfort.

Antimicrobial
An agent that kills or inhibits bacteria, fungi, or viruses.

Inflorescence
A cluster or group of flowers on a plant.

Rhizome
An underground horizontal stem that stores nutrients and can produce shoots and roots.

Poultice
A soft, moist mass of herbs applied externally to relieve soreness and inflammation.

Decoct
To boil plant material to extract active ingredients.

Extract
A concentrated preparation of the active components of a plant.

Herbalism
The practice and study of using plants for medicinal purposes.